PRAISE

"Will resonate with many neurodiverse couples
and relationship counsellors."
TONY ATWOOD, PhD, CLINICAL PSYCHOLOGIST AND CO-AUTHOR OF
NEURODIVERSE RELATIONSHIPS

"A powerful testimony about the ways neurodiverse couples
can cause each other unintentional hurt."
MONA KAY, MSW, PhD, HOST OF
THE NEURODIVERSE LOVE PODCAST

"I read this in one gulp. Wow. This is an important book."
JULIA SCHEERES, NYT BESTSELLING AUTHOR OF *JESUS LAND*

"This unflinching portrait of a marriage will change the way
you look at love... This is a book that needed to be written."
DAVID W. BERNER, AUTHOR OF
DAYLIGHT SAVING TIME: THE POWER OF GROWING OLD

"A vivid, courageous narrative.. and a deep exploration of the
reverberating effects of loss and love."
CAROLINE PAUL, AUTHOR OF *TOUGH BROAD*

"Filled with hope and longing."
MAXINE ASTON, MSc, AUTHOR OF *THE AUTISM COUPLE'S WORKBOOK*

ABOUT THE AUTHOR

Eleanor Vincent is a memoirist and essayist whose work has been recognized by the Feminist Writers' Guild and published in numerous journals and anthologies. Her previous memoir, *Swimming with Maya: A Mother's Story* has twice been on *The New York Times* bestseller list and was a finalist for the Independent Publisher of the Year Award. Her essays have appeared in anthologies by Creative Nonfiction and This I Believe, the literary magazines *580 Split* and *Dorothy Parker's Ashes*, as well as shorter pieces in the *San Francisco Chronicle*, the *Sacramento Bee*, and *Generations Today*. She has an MFA in creative writing from Mills College and is a member of the Author's Guild, the San Francisco Writers Grotto, and Left Margin Lit. She has taught creative nonfiction seminars at Mills College as a visiting writer and been awarded residencies at Hedgebrook, the Vermont Studio Center, and Between the Vines. She lives in Walnut Creek, California.

eleanorvincent.com

DIS CON NEC TED

Portrait *of a* Neurodiverse Marriage

Eleanor Vincent

www.vineleavespress.com

Cover design by Jessica Bell
Interior design by Amie McCracken

For Abby

FOREWORD

With *Disconnected*, Eleanor Vincent has written an immensely personal book about a later-in-life relationship she believed would last forever. She and Lars met, fell deeply in love, and married. It felt like such good fortune. So why does she end up asking for a divorce after only three years?

Eleanor narrates the discovery process that led her from what she imagined her marriage would be to what was realistically possible in her relationship with Lars. Ultimately, what she learned broke her heart.

Eleanor's story echoes many of the stories I hear from the neurodiverse couples around the world with whom I work as a licensed therapist and international coach. These relationships are distinctly different from others, and when the differences are misunderstood or overlooked, problems inevitably emerge.

The challenge is that too often, as Eleanor discovered, these differences and their implications are not generally contextualized as signs of neurodiversity between the partners. Instead, differences are viewed as conscious choices. This is confusing and hurtful for both partners. The underlying fact that each partner is misconstruing the other partner's intent is not obvious to either. Most often, it takes a specialized therapist to help them identify and understand the impact of this bias.

Let's take a minute to describe what neurodiversity means and, of equal importance, what it doesn't mean.

Neurodiversity is a word we use broadly to describe the full range of possible types of brains in our human population, hence *neurotypes*. We refer to the most common neurotype as neurotypical, meaning this is the most prevalent type of brain. Neurotypical does not mean normal, nor does it have any connotation in addition to the frequency with which it occurs among us.

If one partner is neurotypical and the other is not, we call the other partner *neurodivergent*. This simply means that this partner's brain is different from the most commonly occurring neurotypical brain. Among neurodivergences are the diagnoses of Attention Deficit/Hyperactivity Disorder (ADHD), Autism Spectrum Disorder (ASD), dyslexia, Tourette's Syndrome, and several others, as listed in the DSM-5-tr.

A person's neurotype affects the way they experience the world around them as well as the way they process and respond to it. This is where challenges enter a relationship between a neurotypical partner and a neurodivergent partner: each partner expects the other to have a brain like their own. This means they interpret each other's behavior and communication in terms of what it would mean if they did it themselves. And most of the time, such an assessment is not accurate.

Often, a couple commits to a marriage or other partner-ship before having more than a glimmering of the differ-ences between them, and the ones they do recognize are often accounted for as quirky or idiosyncratic aspects of the other partner. Such differences initially seem like parts of the minor compromises and adaptations we expect to make when we choose our partners.

Over time, a clearer picture of differences and divergences arises. It becomes apparent to the couple that their recurrent challenges in understanding each other derive from more than personality or temperament. The fortunate seek care and are correctly guided to understand neurodiversity as the key to unlocking what stands between them.

When I work with couples, I use the analogy of two separate languages. Each partner is fully competent and conversant in their own language. However, they neither understand nor have a guidebook or tutor to help them understand the language of their partner. I use this analogy for several reasons, but most importantly, I use it to underscore that we are talking about differences between two individuals and not pathologizing one or the other as the cause of their challenges.

As we sort these things out in our work together, many couples can bring a new level of compassion and curiosity to their relationship. By employing specific techniques in their communication, couples create more effective methods of connecting two neurotypes. They do this by learning to understand themselves and their own needs as well as their partner and their partner's needs. With this new understanding comes respect and the possibility of accommodation. Couples learn to approach their differences in the spirit of discovery, and, oftentimes, this creates a new spirit of intimacy.

But not always.

When we get to a certain point in our work together, I ask couples to consider the following two questions:

What can I live with?

What can't I live without?

Through this process of discernment, couples can decide whether and how they can stay together, or whether and how they might go their separate ways. Partners must either have an understanding and a plan for how they will continue as a couple, or a destination, a goal, that they can move toward as individuals once they decide to end the relationship. For the sake of each partner's mental health, it is not enough to want to separate without a vision for their next steps.

Sometimes, as in Eleanor's case, the decision to leave was the difficult but necessary path as she considered her situation and what she wanted for her future. Remembering that each couple is unique in their joys and their challenges, let Eleanor show you the path she walked from meeting and falling in love with Lars to the day she decided she needed to set out on her own. Let her strength inspire you if your experience aligns with hers.

Sarah Swenson, LMHC
Seattle, Washington

TheNeurodiverseCouple.com
SarahSwensonLMHC.Substack.com

AUTHOR'S NOTE

Intimate relationships are mysterious. None more so than mine. In the wake of a marriage that lasted three years and nine months to a man with autistic characteristics who refused a diagnosis and only confronted his traits with reluctance, it's impossible to sum things up neatly. My perspective as a neuro-typical woman has been forever changed by my marriage to Lars, a pseudonym I chose to disguise my former husband's identity.

His autistic traits gifted him with amazing abilities and burdened him with perplexing challenges. When he couldn't continue to mask his neurodivergence, the difference in our ways of processing the world led to a bitter cycle of unresolved conflict. It also forced me to reckon with my complex post-traumatic stress disorder (c-PTSD) which overlapped with many of my husband's autistic traits. Ultimately, it caused me to question whether I am neurodivergent myself.

During our marriage, we experienced daily micro-traumas and several more major upheavals: job loss, his and hers cancer diagnoses and treatments, COVID-19, and several rounds of unsuccessful couples counseling. *Disconnected* is the story of how we met and fell in love late in life, and the challenges that drove us apart. Had we chosen to live separately we might have been able to sustain our relationship. But day-to-day life in a high-conflict marriage proved beyond us. Our marriage was an act of courage, but not a fully informed one.

Later, I learned that some estimates show that eighty-five percent of neurodiverse marriages fail. At the time we married, I had no idea.

Some may question whether I have a right to reveal the intimate details of our marriage, or as a neurotypical woman, whether I can fairly describe a man presumed to be neurodivergent. I acknowledge these concerns. "If you meet an autistic person, you've met one autistic person," is a saying I heard often in the support groups we attended. "Don't generalize," was the mantra.

This portrait of Lars is accurate to the way I experienced him. But in no way is this memoir intended to reflect all neurodiverse relationships or all autistic spouses. Thankfully, clinicians are beginning to focus on the special needs of neurodiverse couples. Visit my website for a list of helpful resources.

The autism community is rightly sensitive about neurotypical (NT) people negatively characterizing neurodivergent people or demanding that they fit NT norms. At the same time, NT women in neurodiverse partnerships—and they are mostly women—have a right to describe our experiences and seek support. My charge as I wrote *Disconnected* was to portray our marriage as honestly as I could and to acknowledge my shortcomings and limitations, as well as my husband's. But most of all, to show how much we loved each other and how hard we fought to make our marriage work. It was simply too difficult.

I salute those neurodiverse couples with the patience, fortitude, and emotional intelligence to create workable partnerships. And I offer my heartfelt sympathy to the many couples like Lars and me who ultimately call it quits. The end of our marriage broke my heart. *Disconnected* balances the story of what brought us together with my gradual discovery of the profound differences that ultimately drove us apart. I hope it sheds light on a difficult subject and offers insights to neurodivergent and neurotypical lovers everywhere.

Out of respect for their privacy, I have changed the names and biographical details of some people who appear in these pages.

PROLOGUE

The Lone Ranger uttered few words, but he performed heroic deeds. He wore a mask to hide his identity and rode a white horse named Silver. In my bedroom on Gusty Hill, burrowed under the covers, I used to dream he would ride up to our gray shingle house, stand beneath my window, and call my name.

I would climb out and jump into his arms, rescued at last. He would cradle me tenderly in his arms and shout "Hi-yo, Silver. Away!"

Together we'd gallop over the hill, leaving behind our sad house, my gay father and lesbian mother pretending to be straight, my sister and brother who like me were watched carefully by others in our Pennsylvania town, and my gray cat Pussywillow. I would escape!

Later, on a drive to Cleveland to visit my grandmother, my father played "The William Tell Overture" on the car radio. I recognized it as the opening theme of *The Lone Ranger* TV show. He cranked the radio to top volume. We never heard the siren, but we saw the flashing lights of the Highway Patrol car behind us. Dad glanced in the rear-view mirror, then pulled over and turned down the radio.

"Sir, did you know you were going eighty miles an hour?"

"No, officer," Dad replied, faking humility.

The cop peered at the three of us kids huddled like puppies in the back seat, no seatbelts because they hadn't been invented yet. Mom sat silently in front.

"I'm going to write you a warning ticket, sir. In the future, drive the speed limit."

"I will," Dad said, reaching his hand out the window for the slip of paper.

When the patrol car pulled away, he cranked up the volume again. Lustily, Dad cried, "Hi-yo, Silver. Away!" Gravel pinged the bumper as he spun the car off the shoulder.

We giggled and resumed playing "I Spy," looking forward to stopping at Dad's favorite ice-cream store in Conneaut for chocolate cones.

Hidden identities, secrets and lies, people who went their own way and ignored rules, the operatic fights my parents had, and the way our lives as their children seemed to be an afterthought to their conflicts, made falling in love with a masked man inevitable.

I was predisposed to the strong, silent type, especially one who was smart, courteous, and reserved. I didn't realize the myth of the Lone Ranger held my imagination captive six decades later. On TV, you never got to see him unmasked. In real life, when the mask dropped, my hero was unrecognizable.

At the age of seventy-one, I had married a stranger. If any rescue was going to occur, I'd have to do it myself.

PART I
FALLING IN LOVE

CHAPTER 1
DANCING WITH A COATRACK

"Hey, I'm at the restaurant waiting for you. Let me know your ETA."

My plea lands in my husband's voicemail box, a lonely echo after his greeting.

"Sorry I missed your call," his recording intoned. "Leave a message and I'll get back to you. Until then, as the Dalai Lama says, 'Happiness is determined more by the state of one's mind than by events.'"

"Update me, please," I say, wondering about the state of my own mind.

I want to believe that the gnawing in my belly is only hunger pangs.

That morning, I had asked Lars if he wanted to meet for lunch. He was at his computer, bathed in the green glow of three giant screens. He didn't look up, but he nodded. He mumbled "Yes." I knew that was all I would get.

"Around noon," I said, "Watch for a text, okay?" No response.

I sit in a puddle of light in the restaurant and fiddle with my phone screen. A busboy brings menus, pours water in two glasses, and lays out silverware. Then a server approaches the table.

"Welcome in," she says. "Do you want to wait to order until the other party arrives?"

I'm suspended between appointments with only an hour for lunch.

"No, I'll order now. No telling what he's up to," I say.

I cover my embarrassment with pleasantries, check my texts again: nothing. I phone Lars a second time. He doesn't pick up.

Now, I know he's not coming, but I keep on checking my iPhone, rage simmering in my held breath. I tell myself not to take it personally, gulp for air, trying hard to stay afloat in a familiar sea of neglect.

The waitress sets down my salad. I poke at my shredded lettuce, a few shards of avocado, and the overly grilled shrimp, its burnt edges curling. I tell myself, *Calm down.* But a more insistent voice says, *You're putting up with too much!*

Incidents like this have multiplied like kudzu, crowding out memories of the before time. One fraught afternoon when I had interrupted him in his home office, he pounded his desk so hard that stacks of papers lifted off and fluttered to the floor as he screamed "Leave me alone!" During another meltdown, he growled at me.

After minor disagreements, he would shut down. He would not speak to me for days, even if I addressed him directly. I tiptoed around my husband as if he were a hand grenade with a pulled pin. The atmosphere in our home became so tense that I insisted we start remote sessions with a couple's therapist.

In one of our sessions, Lars told our therapist that maybe he couldn't be a full partner in our relationship because, as he said, "I'm a selfish bastard."

I turned and faced him, my boyish-looking husband with a full head of white hair.

"No, honey, you're not selfish. It's just that your brain is wired differently."

I tried to reassure him that I understood his impenetrable thoughts, his quirks, the ways he left me to fend for myself as if I were still single.

Later, I realized it didn't matter whether he had an undiagnosed autism spectrum disorder or instead was a raging narcissist. The net effect on me was the same.

I've become that person who walks down the street with a big hole in the sidewalk and falls in again and again. Hoping against hope that Lars will be able to reciprocate, I tolerate his neglect, overlook his insults and rudeness, and then when I can't take it anymore, have a meltdown myself. I demand to be recognized as a person with legitimate needs and concerns, I beg to be met. But after three years of our late-in-life marriage, it's getting harder to deny reality: the hole is a bottomless pit.

Lars appears to glory in obtuseness. "I hear you," he says when I try to explain how profoundly alone I feel. He never says, "I'm sorry" or "How can I make it better?" His chief aim is to shut down any conversation that involves a hint of emotion.

He's invented increasingly elaborate ways to disappear, to be absent, to create distance. His work. Important errands. Kiwanis meetings. Reading the latest *New Yorker*. Updating his QuickBooks which can never be interrupted. He's the Houdini of relationships, slipping the bonds of love time after time.

But it didn't begin this way.

⸙

"May I have this dance?"

I was nursing my newly recovered shoulder in the darkened Zydeco dance hall, imagining I'd be a wallflower. I appraised the man standing in front of me.

His shirt looked crisp, as if it had just come from the drycleaners, and he wore his fedora at a rakish angle, a convention of male dancers.

I had seen him at other Zydeco dances before my shoulder injury and noticed that he kissed the back of his partner's hand before escorting her back to her seat, an unusual touch of chivalry. Also, he often sat reading a book before the music began, instead of chatting with the other dancers. I was intrigued by the way he seemed to flout social conventions.

I met his eyes. His smile was like a meteor shower, effervescent.

I projected more confidence than I felt by beaming back and extending my hand.

He took it. Then he led me to the center of the dance floor.

"I'm Lars," he said, looking down at me.

"Hi Lars, I'm Eleanor," I responded, waiting for the music to begin.

I'd been dancing at the Eagles Hall in Alameda, a Bay Area suburb, for fifteen years, but that November night in 2012 was the first time I'd danced in more than ten months. A frozen shoulder had sidelined me. I had missed the music, the camaraderie, and the endorphin high I got from dancing. Zydeco, a dance born in the bayous of southwest Louisiana, serves up a gumbo of happy energy. Many practitioners of the art dance into their eighties and nineties. I imagined Lars was on the younger side, like me, in his sixties.

Zydeco can be intensely physical. I was nervous—would I remember the steps and turns, how would my shoulder hold up, and who was this guy, anyway?

"I haven't seen you in a while," he said.

"I hurt my shoulder, so I took some time off."

"Are you okay now?" He seemed genuinely concerned.

I was wearing a black dress with shoulder straps and a full skirt that flared when I turned, and black dance boots with felt soles that slid over the wooden floor. I spread a gloss of confidence over my fear.

I tried to forget the months of painful physical therapy, the cortisone shots, the disability leave from work.

"Much better," I said. "But please don't spin me too much."

It's easy to cross signals with a new partner. You can miss a beat, or worse, step on each other's feet. It's awkward. Or it can be a joy to glide across the floor in the arms of a skillful leader. I did not know which I was getting when Lars asked me to dance.

As the music began, he took me in his arms.

The accordion chuffed its intense melody, the bass and drums boomed out the rhythm, and the rubboard accented the downbeat.

He held me with a few inches between us, his hand squarely at my mid-back, his palm pushing against mine so that he was easy to follow. I felt guided, secure, in his arms. Dancers have a word for this. It's called "frame." Leaders provide a structure that guides followers safely through the dance allowing them to shine. As Lars moved me skillfully across the floor, I relaxed and surrendered to motion and music.

After starting in closed position, he spun me out in a turn, and to my relief, brought me back in after one spin. He dropped his hand and we moved into open position, where the follower can freelance a bit, still staying in rhythm with the leader. We were in sync!

"That was fun," I said at the end of the song.

"Care for another?"

I nodded. "Yes, please."

The band began a waltz. Lars took me in his arms at a respectful distance but with a confident frame. I closed my eyes and surrendered to the rhythm as we waltzed counterclockwise in a large circle. In time, the movement of the other couples became hypnotic as people dipped and turned and moved into open positions like ice skaters.

The music ended. Lars bowed his head, kissed my hand, and returned me to the table where I had been sitting.

"May I call you sometime?"

I nodded. He handed me a business card.

Helping computers play nice with people for twenty-five years, I read at the bottom.

I dug in my purse and handed him one of my cards. He took it between his thumb and forefinger, bowed slightly, and vanished. Later, other guys I'd danced with before led me onto the dance floor. I hadn't forgotten how to Zydeco!

At the end of the evening, I went to collect my jacket. I was so hot and sweaty, I worried I'd catch a cold, so I wound a scarf around my neck.

Suddenly, Lars appeared in the cloakroom.

"Can I walk you to your car?"

"I'll be fine. Thanks, though," I said.

Alone in the stairwell of the darkened parking garage, I felt a pang. Should I have accepted? Was it possible to be too independent? Or overly standoffish with men?

Zydeco was a safe way to be held and rocked without the illusions of romance or the risk of rejection. My pattern was to see a man's good qualities, fixate on his potential, and overlook warning signs in the flush of infatuation.

Maybe I had become a "relationship anorexic," jargon I had heard in Twelve Step meetings for love addicts, too ambivalent and frightened to let a man get close.

I decided that if Lars did ask me out, I'd take it slow. I'd pay attention. I'd make sure he had the makings of a reliable partner before I got involved. I'd date soberly.

Years later, after our marriage was foundering, I attempted a last-ditch attempt to save it. I suggested to Lars that we meet with a certified autism coach to see if we could untangle our warring neurotypes and learn how to communicate without triggering each other. Barbara held one meeting with us to assess our issues. We filled out a raft of forms to dig into our dynamics. Then she set up meetings with each of us to begin individual coaching. She would not work with us as a couple until she got to know us as individuals.

During our meetings, she drilled me on boundaries, detachment, and self-care. She assigned dozens of articles and book chapters on autism and the special challenges of neurodiverse marriages. I completed the written homework. I tried harder.

"You are dancing with a coatrack," she said in one of our sessions, reminding me of a classic Fred Astaire movie where he grabs a metal coatrack and proceeds to dance with it.

"Yes," I said, "But I still love him."

I knew what she meant, though. There was a long pause before she spoke again.

"You will always have to lead. He will always drag his feet."

Odd, I thought to myself, *because he's such a damn fine dancer!*

Later, despite my pleas, Lars refused to do the homework or continue to meet with Barbara. We were at an impasse. She said she could not coach us as a couple because, she told me, "I don't really know Lars at all."

I felt like saying, "I don't know him either. He's not the same man I married!"

Instead, I told her I was sorry we wouldn't be able to continue to work with her as a couple. I had to face the truth: I couldn't save our marriage alone. It would take many more months—and a six-week stay in Europe by myself—before I summoned the courage to step out on my own.

When hope was truly lost, I revisited how we had come together. I wanted to make sense of my inability to see how deep our differences were. I needed to understand why I had married a man I had believed was my best friend but who had morphed into a silent, stony enigma. I traveled back to our beginnings, to all that drew us together.

CHAPTER 2
THE DATING GAME

A week after I met Lars at the Eagles Club in the fall of 2012, I received a message from him on LinkedIn. He didn't text, or phone, or ask to friend me on Facebook. Instead, he gave me a window into his work history, his network, and his interests: Kiwanis International (he was a long-term member), The Commonwealth Club, City Arts and Lectures.

It was a far cry from the exaggerated profiles I used to scroll through on Match.com or e-Harmony. I'd tried internet dating for several years and given up. Coffee dates with that many frogs pretending to be princes were a waste of time!

In his message, Lars asked if I'd read the latest book by Malcolm Gladwell and if I subscribed to *The New Yorker*. Regretfully, no, I told him. He must have been thinking about what I'd said about being a writer the night we met. He was trying to connect.

Several days passed. I contemplated calling Lars but decided against it. At sixty-four, I'd been divorced for almost thirty years. I had had several serious partners and some rough breakups. I'd been through the dating mill, and I wasn't looking for drama. Too much hurt made me shy away, like a highly strung horse when a new rider approaches. A reliance on healthy boundaries provided an excuse not to reach out after my initial response to his message.

A few days later, he called me. I felt a little flutter when I saw his name on my phone screen. I was pleased that he was motivated enough to take the initiative.

We chatted about the Zydeco dance scene and our work, and then he mentioned that he was a subscriber to one of the community theaters in Berkeley.

"I have tickets for Wednesday night, care to join me?"

I hesitated. How was I going to fit dating a new man into my already packed schedule?

"That's nice of you, Lars. I'm super busy right now and mid-week is not the best time for me. How about a weekend activity?"

We discussed hiking, or dinner and a movie, but my mind kept darting off to work deadlines, my writing commitments, making time for family and friends.

I stood up, clutching the phone in my hand. I couldn't say yes. I liked my straight jacket of chores. It comforted me. It made me feel I knew what was coming next. With this new man, like an intriguing bauble on a very high shelf, I had no idea what would happen if I took a chance. If experience was any guide, he wouldn't turn out to be as shiny and enticing as he currently appeared.

"I have to go," I said, "Busy day tomorrow. Thanks for calling."

"I'll see you at Eagles on Friday," he said. "Maybe we can settle on a date then."

I swiped off my phone screen and released a long-held sigh. My whooshing breath felt as if I was in an old-school Western movie where the hero's loneliness is symbolized by a puff of wind blowing tumbleweed across a desolate plain.

I looked around at my kitchen, at the knives in the dish drainer, the striped cotton dish towel, the African violet on the window ledge, the photos of my granddaughter on the wall by the sink. *Okay*, I said to myself. *You're alone. But are you lonely?*

"Lonely older woman" is such a tired trope. I preferred to see myself as a vibrant seasoned professional. I had often asked myself what I was willing to sacrifice for peace of mind and career success. I knew "having it all" was a bald-faced lie. A friend had told me years ago that a woman can have two of three: a man, children, or a great job. I had the great job, and the kids, one still standing after my daughter Maya's death in a horse-riding accident twenty years earlier. I still had my younger daughter, Greta, her husband, and a gorgeous grand-daughter. But the man? That eluded me.

Lars touched me with his reticence, his politeness. Courtly manners went a long way with me; I was unaccustomed to being handled so carefully. On top of that, he was an awesome dancer. Any woman in the Zydeco scene will tell you that finding a partner like Lars is like finding the pony in the pile of manure and being presented with the Hope Diamond in the same moment. My outrageous good luck!

But three decades with on-again, off-again boyfriends had left its imprint. Did I want to risk my precious solitude for a dazzling smile and a few slick dance moves?

My orange tabby cat, Saffron, rubbed my ankles, begging for food. I reached down to scratch his ears. Through an unforeseen miracle (and an implanted chip) he had been returned to me after running away when I first moved to Oakland. He was scarred and beaten up from his six years on the road, the Jack Kerouac of cats. His paw pads were worn away and his scrawny frame bespoke his years of living untended, scrounging for handouts.

"Okay, mister, you're my number one," I crooned.

I sealed the deal with a fresh helping of kibble, and Saffron nuzzled into his bowl, purring like a toy train.

CHAPTER 3
CANDLELIGHT

My cheeks burned in the darkened theater, and the plush seat scratched my back. Lars and I had agreed to see *The Sessions*, a daring choice for a first date. I snuck a glance at him, but he was focused on the screen. I shifted in my seat.

The movie was about a man with polio who lives in an iron lung, based on the real-life disability activist Mark O'Brien. He hires a sex surrogate because he wants to experience touch and sexual arousal, a form of connection he hungers for. Helen Hunt plays the sex worker, Cheryl, who offers more than just sex. Understanding. Empathy. Tenderness.

To leap from being dance partners to a display of explicit onscreen sex was, well, awkward. Yet I was moved by the ways these strangers found comfort in each other's arms.

I once dated a man who was crippled on one side. He'd taken a bullet to the right side of his head, and so he walked like a turning wheel, lifting his left side, heaving it in an arc to keep moving forward. I fell in love with Mike. He was a poet and a survivor.

In ways no one else had, he "got" me. Mike saw all the ways I was emotionally crippled. My heart was like a turning wheel, too; partly frozen, so that I had to jerk it along to keep moving forward. As a child, I had to pretend to be tough to survive emotional and physical abuse. My trust was always partial, half-hearted, testing to see if I could find anyone I could rely on. I trusted Mike because his wounds were visible, and he wore them bravely, without apology. I had spent a lifetime hiding my tender, vulnerable side. He made it safe for me to emerge.

Watching *The Sessions* made me remember Mike and our brief, intense affair. It also made me wonder about Lars and me, whether we'd have sex.

That night we kissed for the first time, a mixture of affection and restrained passion. After that, Lars began texting me erotic haiku. This is promising, I thought; he has a poetic bent.

***

Three days before Christmas, Lars appeared at my home uninvited. When I opened the door, he handed me a huge bouquet of bright flowers.

"They're lovely," I said. "Any special reason?"

"They made me think of you," he said. "Maybe I was just looking for an excuse to see you ..." He trailed off.

"Come in," I said, opening the door wider.

He was wearing a brown fedora and his yellow Nepalese scarf.

I searched his face as he unwound his scarf and took off his jacket. He was handsome in a tailored way, with silver hair, a firm jaw, regular features, and blue-gray eyes, a head taller than me. When asked where he was from, he'd always answer that he was born in Oslo. He'd never say he was Norwegian. Because, the truth was, that he had left his birth country at the age of two and become a naturalized American citizen when he was a senior in high school. He had gone to grade school in the Midwest and then moved with his family to the Manhattan suburbs. But he rarely mentioned those places.

Over time, I understood that he liked being exotic, always a little mysterious. Lars never wanted to appear ordinary; he read extraordinarily difficult science and philosophy books, never novels, claiming he couldn't understand the emotions underlying the stories.

He took off the fedora and placed it reverently on the desk by the front door. I'd discovered that he had an extensive collection of hats that he treasured.

When I'd cut the flower stems and arranged them in a vase, I busied myself making tea. This was something we had in common—we were both tea drinkers, preferring the more expensive loose tea brands. At last, we settled on my couch. I tried to appear casual.

"You surprised me," I admitted. "After I didn't hear from you this week, I figured you were busy for the holidays."

Lars only smiled and sipped his tea. "Just busy at work," he said.

My tree had been up and decorated since the day after Thanksgiving. I'd already shipped presents to my brother and sister in Ohio and had done the bulk of the Christmas shopping for my daughter Greta and her family. I loved getting presents. I also loved giving them. Gifts were an expression of love, an act of care and generosity.

"I have a little gift for you," I said, remembering the present in its tastefully wrapped box. I had purchased it at a high-end home goods store in my neighborhood after carefully considering what to buy for a man I didn't know all that well.

Lars raised one bushy eyebrow. I rose and went to retrieve his gift from beneath the tree. He looked suspended between surprise and muted delight.

He turned the small box in his hands, then held it up and shook it.

I put a hand on his arm. "Don't do that," I warned. "It's breakable."

"What can it be?" I couldn't tell if he was mocking me, or genuinely curious.

He removed the wrapping methodically, careful not to tear the paper. He slit the gold sticker on the box with his thumbnail and removed his gift, studying it carefully. Then he looked at me with a puzzled expression on his face.

"It's Mercury glass," I explained. "Antique. For holding a votive candle."

"Why?"

I hesitated. Was he joking?

"It's meant to be romantic, you know, for the bedside table."

He stared at me with a blank expression.

"Mood lighting," I said. "In case, if we should, you know, decide...to make love..."

My voice drifted off. My cheeks glowed with embarrassment.

Lars smiled. But his eyes told me that either he didn't get it, or he didn't believe me. Which was it?

"Oh," he said. "That didn't occur to me. About the candle, I mean."

The erotic Japanese haiku he'd been texting me each morning showed that he had thought about sex. But my reciprocal romantic gesture had fallen flat. Lars did not associate antique candle holders with candlelight next to a bed, turned-down covers, or the slip of lingerie to the floor. I began to understand why he never read novels.

"Well, thank you," he said, too heartily.

"There's a candle and some matches too," I said.

He felt around in the box, found the other items, and then tucked the Mercury glass holder back on its bed of tissue paper and closed the box.

I was mortified. I felt as if I'd stuck my neck out way farther than I'd meant to, tipped my hand too soon, and sent an invitation that went unrecognized and thus, unreceived.

There's a scene in *Zorba the Greek* where Anthony Quinn tells a young Alan Bates, that if a woman calls a man to her bed, it's a sin not to go.

The Alan Bates character is afraid to sleep with the beautiful widow played by Irene Pappas. But Zorba's encouragement pushes him to take a chance, and a steamy affair follows.

At that moment, I wished for my own personal Zorba. Alas, no such exuberant Greek existed in my orbit! And I was still too early in my relationship with Lars to read the tea leaves.

Was he clueless about the subtleties of seduction? Or was something more at play?

In the time I'd known him, I had seen signs of Asperger's syndrome: difficulty with eye contact, skimming over or avoiding emotional topics, obsessive focus on his work. I'd read about the characteristics of autism-1, considered high functioning. When I worked in information technology at a previous job, I'd encountered computer nerds who were gifted but also difficult. They were brilliant, obsessive, and possibly on the autism spectrum; one of them had a tantrum in the office and screamed at a colleague, then slammed his office door so hard we cubicle-dwellers flinched.

I had a "Psychology Today" vision of Asperger's syndrome. The newer terminology referred to autistic people as being "neurodivergent" or "neuroatypical."

I reasoned to myself, who is typical? Surely not me, a highly sensitive abuse survivor and bereaved mother with PTSD and complex grief who jumps every time a door slams and can't stand the sound of anyone chewing. I have everything—IBS, misophonia, migraines, sleep disturbance. Every somatic symptom you've possibly never even heard of. Who was I to judge?

I passed off his puzzlement over my gift as general male clue-lessness.

Maybe Lars was just a garden-variety guy with little aware-ness of his feelings. Maybe he was a narcissist, a member of the male species I attracted like flies to honey.

We finished our tea. I said I had some last-minute shopping to do, and Lars offered to go with me. My idea of hell is a shop-ping center a few days before Christmas, closely followed by being in a crowd waiting in line for the Tomorrow Land ride at Disneyland. I told him about my dread, but he was unphased.

"It will be fun," he promised.

He was jolly as we got in his Prius and headed for the Barnes and Noble mega-store in Emeryville. He got us there by taking shortcuts I'd never discovered and avoiding a traffic jam on Highway 80. As we rode the escalator up to the children's book section, I scanned the crowded store anxiously, already over-whelmed by the choices, the other shoppers browsing in the book aisles, coming toward us in noisy groups on the down escalator.

Lars put a hand on my back and guided me off the escalator, heading purposefully toward the kids' books. Within half an hour I had several colorful picture books, two puzzles, and some small notebooks and colored pencils for my granddaughter. I'd never shopped so efficiently in my life. He was right. It *was* fun.

An hour later we stood in my front hall. Lars gave me a kiss goodnight. It was tender and sweet, full of promise. I wondered if perhaps I had misjudged him, his bafflement about the candle holder, his lack of sincere gratitude, his matter-of-fact return of the gift to its box.

"See you at Eagles," he said. "There's a great band next weekend."

And then he was gone. When I returned to my living room I found the gift in its box, the wrapping paper tucked neatly beside it on my couch. I considered texting him, but something told me not to. We had crossed wires. There was no point in calling him back to retrieve a gift he didn't understand and likely didn't want.

Later, I would look back at that night. If our relationship had been a game of Clue, it should have been obvious: Colonel Mustard in the living room with a candlestick.

But no crimes had been committed—yet—and I remained blissfully clueless.

CHAPTER 4
LOVE AND DEATH

For Valentine's Day, Lars asked me out to dinner at a little Italian place he knew about.

To prepare for a romantic evening, I got a manicure and had my hair styled. I put on my sexiest top.

"You look beautiful," Lars said when he picked me up.

"Thanks," I said and kissed him on the cheek.

In the dimly lit restaurant, we traded bites of pasta and shared a decadent chocolate dessert. Later, I gave him a Valentine's card that showed a teacup with a teabag labeled "OCD" (that's the girl) and a coffee cup (the boy) with a stir stick labeled "Anxiety." The two cups are nestled side by side and the girl cup is smiling and batting her painted eyelashes at the boy cup. The caption reads, "We go together like a couple of co-morbid psychiatric disorders."

Lars barely cracked a smile.

He was a mystery. I was drawn to his intelligence, and a quality of tenderness in the way he held me when we danced, always opened doors for me, and carried bags when we went shopping. He was polite, solicitous, even gallant. It was sweet and old-fashioned. I loved his scent of clean shirts and an essential oil he wore called Night Rain that was musky, and how his palms were always dry and never clammy. It finally hit me: *I am falling in love.*

We'd been dating for almost three months, and we still hadn't done the deed. I was grateful he wasn't pushing me, but at the same time wondering why he wasn't more focused on getting me into bed. We had some thrilling make-out sessions, so I wondered why we both hesitated. Part of me still lingered in the 1950s and '60s when men were supposed to take the lead and it was a "good girl's" job to hold them at bay. My Catholic upbringing went deep.

I decided on a strategy of watchful waiting. Lars had a low-key way of responding to things. His emotions seemed to range from detachment to mild interest.

One evening after we'd gone out to a movie, he kissed me tenderly at the door, and I kissed back more passionately than before. I thought he might stiffen and pull away but instead, he met me with equal ardor, and we melted together.

After we released our embrace, Lars looked at me with an expression I didn't know how to interpret. He seemed puzzled, even bashful.

"I'll call you soon," he said, and then he was gone.

I leaned against the door for a moment, then turned and deadbolted it. Later, snuggled in bed, I fretted. I didn't want to jump in too soon or blunder into an ill-fated affair, but I knew that, ultimately, desire would win out over doubt.

The old days were so much easier—just leap into bed and worry about it afterward—but I didn't want to go down the familiar path of infatuation, hasty commitment, regret, and breakup. I was looking for something more, for someone who could be a real partner.

I once had a therapist who reminded me that there are six people in an intimate relationship—the couple and both sets of parents. Our parents are our first loves and our most important role models. This might explain why I usually fell for handsome narcissists who were of the "bad boy" or artistic variety: that described my father to a T.

Dad was a charismatic drama professor and actor, beloved by his students, and known for his idiosyncratic techniques as a theater director. He once put a pine board down a student's pants and kicked him across the stage to teach him proper posture.

Putting it charitably, he was not a patient man. His raging outbursts terrified me. As his outspoken oldest child, I was a girl with a target on her back.

But as he aged, and dementia set in, he gradually became more tolerant. Suddenly, he overflowed with endearments. His phone messages were sprinkled with "dear hearts" and "darlings," and his conversations became odes to the virtues of his three children.

"Who *is* that man?" My sister Tess and I would commiserate after our calls with Dad.

He had become a softer version of his more abrasive younger self. Over time, I began to trust the newer version. I liked demented, affectionate ninety-three-year-old Dad a whole lot better.

By then, he had been a resident of the Actor's Fund Home in Englewood New Jersey for ten years. The home was a welcoming place where former Actors Equity members could shelter in old age. Dad had survived colon cancer surgery and a broken hip. On top of that, he had emphysema from years of smoking. Lately, his dementia had worsened. In mid-February of 2013, we got the call: Dad was gravely ill. Could we come?

Walking down the corridor to my father's room, my nose puckered with a casserole of scents: disinfectant, Lemon Pledge, musty laundry, and something indefinable, the smell of funk, of approaching death.

Some residents sat in wheelchairs in the hall. Each day when we arrived, I would wave to them, and if there was a flicker of a response, say hello.

I'd look at them and stare into my imagined future, my hair frizzy, wrinkles etched on the map of my cheeks, my skin dry as paper, my neck in folds like a turkey wattle. I couldn't compute, so I hurried on.

In Dad's room, my brother and sister stood on either side of his bed. He was gasping for air, panicking, ripping the oxygen lines out of his nose, trying to throw his leg over the bed rail to escape his sweaty nest of tangled sheets.

My once all-powerful father undone by his failing lungs, gasped like a child with croup, a scared, cowering child. Except that he was my *father*, not a child. He was an old man dying of emphysema in broad fucking daylight, his middle-aged children as witnesses.

My sister made way for me and went to sit at the foot of the bed.

Looking down at him, his gaping toothless mouth, his gigantic elf ears, his watery blue eyes I had no choice. I had to forgive. He was helpless, mortal.

But when I was ten he was a God who roared and screamed, who threatened to cut off my ears if I spilled my milk, who once told me my rear end stuck out like a bustle, and later that same day, after I arrived home late for dinner, whipped my bare legs with a branch he pulled off our maple tree, the cutting sound as it whistled through the air, the briny sting of my blood, the welts rising on the backs of my thighs below my khaki shorts right out there on our front sidewalk where anyone could see. He was a master of humiliation. My father. Now a husk, a body struggling to draw breath, no longer an object of terror.

"It's Ellie, Dad," I said. I stroked his hair. "It's okay," I lied. "It's going to be okay."

His eyes swirled towards me, pleading.

"You are so lovely. So lovely," he repeated over and over as I held his hand. I tried to absorb his words without breaking into tears, without remembering the ten-year-old girl with welts on her legs, without feeling the weight of his cruelties.

Without warning, Dad grabbed the bedrail and struggled upright.

"I have to get out of here!" He wheezed.

As gently as I could, I pushed his shoulders down.

"We're trying to help you get out of here, Dad," I said, by which I meant, out of your failing body, out of this suffering. "But you have to stay in bed."

His shoulder blades were delicate as sparrow's bones. My brother and I locked eyes across our father's prone body.

"He needs more medication," I said.

My sister ran to the nurse's station to beg for more tranquilizers.

Tim and I stood like military guards on either side of Dad's bed.

The day was interminable. The flailing, the gasping, the intense locked-eyed stares, trying to let my father know he was not alone, we would not abandon him, he was loved despite everything, more loved than I could ever say.

That afternoon, I left and made it as far as the hall outside his door. There I put my forehead against the cool tile wall and sobbed.

"I got it all backward," Dad told Tim while I was out in the hall.

I didn't know for sure what he meant, but I wanted to believe my father knew that his stinging words and raging blows had all been a terrible mistake, a symptom of PTSD from his time in Guam and Iwo Jima during the war. That in our family, he and I were the most alike: the neediest, the most hyperbolic, the most fearful, the ones most likely to deflect with humor and defend with sarcasm. I was his mirror image.

I asked Tim what Dad meant.

"I'm not sure," he said, "He just kept saying it over and over."

That night, I phoned Lars to give him an update. Up until then, I had said little about my family dynamics, only that I had a difficult relationship with my father. When I told him about my grief and how much my father was suffering, his response was rote but sympathetic.

"It sounds rough," he said.

"It's hellish," I responded. "But at the same time, I'm glad I came."

Lars said he'd pick me up at the San Francisco airport, and that he was eager for me to come home. I told him I'd worn a skirt and sweater he had given me as a gift, and that my father had complimented me on it.

"You have very good taste," I told Lars, knowing that would please him.

Two days later the three of us left. Dad was medicated and confused. He kept asking if we were coming back. Tim assured him that he would be back in a few weeks. When it was my turn, I went to his bedside and squeezed my father's hand.

"Bye, Daddy," I said. "Behave yourself. Do what the nurses tell you."

He squeezed my hand in response. I had a plane to catch, a life calling me home. Otherwise, I would have lingered. I patted his cheek, turned on my heel, and walked away.

CHAPTER 5
EMERGENCY SEX

Amid my father's dying, life went on. I had my nine-to-five job editing clinical content for a new physician website my employer was building; Lars and I were negotiating when, or whether, we would have sex; and at the same moment my memoir about the death of my older daughter, *Swimming with Maya,* had been reissued in paperback and e-book.

I did my work as an author and promoted the book. My new website went live. My publisher's publicity campaign unfurled. And I was due in Phoenix for a promotional event in under a week. After that, Lars and I planned to go away for a weekend together. We had been dating for three months; I finally felt okay about moving forward.

I had reserved a cottage in the seaside town of Bolinas on the Northern California coast for the last weekend in February. But as the day grew closer, I felt overwhelmed. I realized that didn't have the emotional bandwidth for a romantic weekend.

"I need to cancel our trip," I told Lars in a phone call. "I've got too much going on."

It was more than I could bear to think about packing a suitcase, arranging cat care, leaving piles of unfinished work on my desk at home and at the office, and waiting for a phone call telling me that my father had died.

"I'm sorry," I said. "I imagine you're disappointed."

He said nothing but I could hear tension in his silence.

"Okay, I'll talk to you later," I said.

I paused hoping he would respond. But he still did not answer me, so I hung up.

As the week wore on, I texted my apologies. I emailed. I phoned and left voice mails but I heard nothing.

I began to question if I had the strength for this. "He may be too high maintenance," I mused in my journal. I knew that I had been through too much to bend myself into a pretzel to please a man, especially one who couldn't find a few words to respond, even if they were just "I need some space" or "I'm upset." Something.

I'm not sure why I was so patient with Lars. I'd be ready to give up on him, and then he'd do or say something endearing, and I'd find myself wanting to be with him. Or I'd see him at the Eagles Hall, and we'd dance, and the feel of his solidity, his broad shoulders, his barrel chest would give me a sense of physical security. Despite his quirks, I trusted Lars. His mysterious calmness soothed me.

Finally, I asked him over to work things out. I suggested we walk and talk first, with tea to follow. I was pleased when he agreed and appeared at my door.

We wound up the hills near my house, higher and higher into the urban forest of the Piedmont Community Park. Perhaps it was foolish to attempt logic with him. I had begun to see that if he felt slighted, or ignored, or became disappointed, he sulked with the ferocity of a stymied toddler.

I promised that once my book promotion eased, we'd reschedule our trip to Bolinas. I got nowhere. He was implacable.

In utter frustration, I faced him and began pounding on his chest on the corner of Crocker and LaSalle Avenues. "Let me in! Let me in!"

I hammered on his chest with closed fists, oblivious to passersby.

Lars stared down at me impassively as a statue.

"Colloidal suspension," he said at last, "Do you know what that is?"

"No idea," I replied, wondering how I managed to be standing on the sidewalk pounding on the chest of Bill Nye the Science Guy.

With less emotional affect than a passing cloud, Lars explained interface and colloid science as propounded by Italian chemist Francesco Selmi in excruciating detail. I took him to mean that he was as solid as concrete. There was further discussion of ions and molecules, and I later came to understand that colloids fall into multiple categories including gasses and liquids, so the concrete analogy didn't really apply. It didn't matter: Lars was immovable.

As we wended our way down Wildwood Avenue he repeated, "I want to go to Bolinas! I want to go to Bolinas," in broken record cadence, pumping his arms up and down like a four-year-old about to unleash a sulfurous tantrum.

I went mute. I had to find a way to redirect this sixty-year-old toddler.

Once we got home, I put on water for tea. I was keyed up tight as a jack in the box, desperate to find some compromise, to help us move forward.

Lars stood by the window, looking out over the trees over-topping Lakeshore Avenue. A bluish-black dusk as soft as velvet began to enfold the apartment. I realized I had to give Lars something tangible. Words weren't going to be enough.

I went up behind him and put my arms around his waist. I rubbed my cheek against his broad back. His wool sweater scratched my skin.

"Let's have Bolinas right here," I said.

I faced the gathering darkness in my windows, and half turned away from Lars, and my mind was a mirror for my stance in the room. I half knew what I was saying, but half denied it just like the half-darkness enveloping my deck. I meant let's have sex. That's what staying in a rented cottage by the sea implies. It means we are ready for the next step, the leap into the unknown of fulfilled passion. It might be wonderful. It might be a disaster. I sensed that nothing would placate Lars but that. And I didn't want to live in suspense for another minute.

"We need to have emergency sex," I said. "Right now."

I turned to face him; he looked down into my eyes. That morning, the call about Dad had finally come. Tim said our father had died just before dawn, with his favorite nurse at his bedside. I immediately sat down and wrote a first draft of my father's obituary and sent it to my brother. But I proceeded with my day and reconnecting with Lars.

I had all the feelings you get even after an expected death: the immensity of the heartbreak, the mystery of that person I had loved and hated, and forgiven so much, vanishing from the earth. Yet here I stood with Lars, a man who seemed so oppo-site to my combustible father; he was equally mysterious to me, but alive, looking into my eyes.

I slid my arms around his neck, and he bent to kiss me, his breath warm on my face, his lips a soft shock against mine. After all the hard words, we melted into one another, the atoms, ions, and molecules dissolving in shared heat. The colloidal particles melted into an intoxicating mashup of new love and urgent desire.

I took his hand and led him into my bedroom. I turned down the duvet and stacked throw pillows on a nearby chair. Then I lit a votive candle and set it on my bookshelf. If he didn't know the purpose of candlelight before, now was his chance.

Lars unbuttoned my blouse, and I let it fall to the floor. Then I snuggled against him and listened as his heart galloped in his chest.

There's a scene in the movie *Big* where Tom Hanks, a twelve-year-old trapped in an adult body, first encounters a woman's breast. He runs his fingers around its curves, exploring reverently. That was how Lars touched me, gently at first, with a sense of wonder, and then urgently, pulling off my clothes.

I climbed into bed, and he slid in after me, encircling me in his arms, kissing my neck, and then my breasts, sliding one hand between my thighs. As he inched his way down my belly, I put my hand on his hair and tugged. He lifted his head and looked at me.

"Is this okay?"

"It's perfect," I said. "Don't let me interrupt you."

He gave me the same dazzling smile I had seen the night we met.

"Kiss, please," I said, and he slid himself up along my torso. He covered my face with kisses and when our lips met, lingered there, gently stroking me as I grew wet. I had lubricant in the bedside table, but we weren't going to need it. I had worried that he might lose his erection, and when I told him this, he laughed.

"It's just hydraulics," he said. "Don't worry."

I guided him inside me and then begged for him to be still.

"Push," I said, "Then, stay."

He followed my instructions precisely with just the right amount of pressure, holding steady as I pulsed around him, merging with his body. I groaned.

"Am I hurting you?"

"No silly, you're making me come."

When I gave permission to move, he joined me in a dance more intricate and compelling than any moves he had led on the dance floor. Sweaty and satisfied, I lay in his arms afterward, stroking his chest. The colloidal suspension—his analog for frozen feelings—had dissolved, the web of hesitation we had been caught in for three long months gave way.

"How was that?" I asked.

"Nice," he said.

I pushed up on my elbow and looked at him, incredulous.

"Nice? I'm moaning in ecstasy and you're telling me it was *nice*?"

To me, nice is a word you use to describe a pleasing cup of tea, not love making with your new partner.

But Lars only smiled. "What's important is that you enjoyed it."

"I loved it!"

He smiled and pulled me to him, and I lay against his chest, synchronizing my breath with his. Moments later I felt his leg twitch, and he disappeared into sleep.

CHAPTER 6
LEARNING HIS BODY

One Sunday afternoon a few weeks after we had become lovers, Lars and I were lying in his bed talking, and the topic turned to physical attraction.

"I imagine that I am not your physical type," he said.

Hanging near the bed was a wooden bar holding his neatly pressed shirts on plastic hangers. I studied it, partly to avoid looking at the jumble of random items and dust bunnies in his room, and partly to give myself time to parse my words.

"You're right," I said after a pregnant pause where I'd carefully considered the stripes and checks, the blues and greens, the extraordinarily precise way those shirts hung in a row.

Earlier in my life, if I had seen Lars in a bar or at a dance, I might have been arrested by his smile, or his propensity for wearing expensive fedoras, but his big body would have been a turn-off. Yet here I was lying next to him naked, my chest pressed against his, our bellies touching, skin pushing against skin. What had happened?

I'd been married to two extraordinarily handsome men and in the wake of two divorces, dated some even better-looking ones. Bit by bit, year by year, I discovered that many handsome men are selfish bastards. I hate to generalize but I feel that most women of a certain age will back me up on this.

So, when Lars invited me to dance that night in 2012, and when he pulled me towards him, and his round Santa Claus belly pressed against my midriff, instead of being repulsed I found it comforting. It was as if he was touching me without touching, without intruding on my personal space. His physical heft made me feel safe.

Now, I confessed what was true: Lars was *not* my type. But by then I'd learned to back away from men who were.

When I said, "You're right," I swallowed hard, wondering how he would take this. I continued to study the shirts, picturing Lars's body in them, clothed.

"Yeah," he finally said, "I guess there's no accounting for taste."

"The men that I thought were my physical type have turned out to be jerks," I said.

I was owning up to my shallow self, that woman who kept falling in love with men like her father, fussy men who cared way too much about their images, who primped, who turned out to be narcissists, some of them even abusive. I didn't say any of this. Instead, I moved closer and felt his warmth leaching into my body. I believed that, at long last, I had found genuine love.

Dad's memorial service was set for the first weekend in June at the Actor's Fund Home in Englewood. I asked Lars to fly to New Jersey with me. I didn't want to be the only one of us three siblings to face the day with no partner by my side. He readily agreed. He even bought a navy-blue suit for the occasion.

I discovered that Lars was as good at traveling as he was at shopping. Getting checked in at the airport, disposing of luggage, boarding, and finding a seat, all things I find nerve-wracking, went smoothly. The flight was a breeze.

The first hint of awkwardness arose when we arrived at the airport in Newark. My brother and his wife were going to pick us up. No one in my family had met Lars. Moments before we were due to meet Tim and his wife Alyssa outside baggage claim, my heart fluttered.

"My brother is ... umm ... very well organized," I said between held breaths. "He has an executive streak."

My brother was the CEO of a successful business, a company he had founded thirty-five years before, and a powerhouse in the Midwest. He had an iPhone growing out of his ear with a raft of clients on speed dial.

I checked Lars's expression to see how this was landing. His face was neutral, almost blank. *He's not getting it*, I thought.

"He can be tightly wound," I said, then backtracked. "I mean, you'll like him and everything, he's very likable. He just has strong views."

"Is that like anyone we know?" Lars asked slyly.

"Gosh, I can't imagine who," I said, linking my arm with his.

We walked through the airport toward the escalator down to baggage claim. Little kids dragged carry-on suitcases with red and blue Mickey Mouse faces while Moms and Dads hurried them along. The smell of See's candy and human funk permeated the air.

I desperately wanted Lars and Tim to like each other, and it suddenly hit me that I was dropping Lars into the deep end of the pool without a life jacket. I was about to submerge him in my family dynamics and realized I hadn't prepared him for what my brother ironically called "the sparkling Vincent personality."

I hustled to make up for lost time.

"Tim was Dad's favorite," I said. "He was the baby of the family, and the story goes that my parents never slept together again after he was born."

Lars shot me a look of mild alarm.

"They were waiting for their boy..." I said, although there was so much more buried in that revelation. I couldn't even imagine explaining. *You see, once upon a time, two people who desperately needed to pass as straight in the late 1940s decided to get married even though they both knew they were gay ...* I couldn't possibly say this.

I swallowed. There was no way to prepare Lars to meet my family. I was barely prepared myself, and I *knew* them, I knew the history the way a fish knows water. It was pretty much unspeakable, even the long version. The short version was incomprehensible.

Maybe it was then that I finally got it: I didn't suffer from writer's block. I had life block. How could I ever give voice, select words, and create order out of the chaos that had been my childhood? The raw material I had to work with was like a vat of unset concrete—mushy, yet heavy—and I would never be able to get it to set up.

I dodged around the family in front of us, letting go of Lars's arm. Suddenly, I let go of my anxiety too. He was just going to have to dive in. I couldn't protect him. All I could do was go through the discovery with him and see what we could learn.

I felt immense gratitude toward Lars. He was brave. It might be naïve bravery, uninformed courage, but that didn't make it any less laudable. He strode toward baggage claim, about to pluck our bags off the carousel, about to fall straight into the deep end.

Lars and Tim were the same age. With a similar matter-of-fact approach, they hit it off immediately. They loaded our luggage in the car, and Tim piloted us to the Hilton Express where we were staying.

My sister Tess and her husband Adam had already checked in. Once everyone had unpacked, we gathered in the hotel dining room. All we'd had on the flight was some ginger ale and a pack of peanuts. I scanned the menu like a crazed hyena.

"I reserved a table at Dad's favorite restaurant, Lattanzi, for tomorrow night," Tim said. He'd also gotten tickets to "Lucky Boy," the last play Nora Ephron wrote, which had just opened on Broadway.

I'd never been to a Broadway show before; I was thrilled at the prospect.

"So, what do you do, Lars?"

My sister turned to my beloved expectantly.

"I help computers play nice with people," Lars said.

Tess's face went blank as a sheet of paper.

The waitress set down our salads.

"He's a computer consultant," I explained. "Macs, PCs, iPhone issues, databases."

Tim's face lit up. He launched into some network issues he was trying to troubleshoot. He and Lars both had foamy dark beers by their plates; my brother-in-law Adam was drinking a Coke. The ladies all had iced tea. I swirled the ice in my glass with a long spoon, dunking my lemon slices.

So far, no one had said anything awkward or off-putting, and I began to relax.

My sister poked her fork in the depths of her salad as if she was looking for something.

"So where does your family live, Lars?"

I felt him stiffen as if his shirt sleeve had suddenly grown a coat of starch.

"In New York," he said. "Rye."

This was only an hour drive from where we were sitting. I had already argued with Lars about his very firm plans not to see his parents or his sister. His staunch insistence on maintaining distance from his family mystified me.

Tim raised an eyebrow. Tess kept going.

"Oh, did you grow up there?"

"I was born in Oslo," Lars said, leaving it open-ended as if he had lived in Norway most of his life.

Both my sibs stared at him. Adam set down his Coke. Alyssa wiped her lips with her napkin.

"His parents emigrated when he was two," I explained. I knew Lars wanted to keep the mystery going but I wasn't having it.

"We lived in the Midwest when I was in grade school," he said. "When my dad got a new job with a better company we moved."

Lars had this way of skipping things, of making everything seem so cut and dried, as if, of course, his Norwegian parents would have wound up in Rye. And he would have been just a normal high school kid. All far from true.

During the second month of our courtship, Lars told me his mother had attempted suicide. He had said this casually, leaning back against my couch cushions.

"I'm so sorry," I said. "That must have been hard for you."

He shrugged. "Not really," he had said.

I was stunned. My mind had immediately swung into high gear.

"Have you ever ... I mean did you ever think about killing yourself?"

Lars had appraised me for a minute. He shook his head. "No, but I had a serious depression after my second marriage ended."

Somehow, we kept on. I learned he had gone to therapy, mostly a waste of time, he had said, although he learned some helpful behavioral tricks. He was better he said. I made a mental note: red flag, but, still, I was falling in love. Now, more months in, I forced myself back to the moment, to the faux wood table, my salad, and iced tea.

I nudged Lars with my thigh, and he nudged back.

"Will you see your family while you're here?" This from my sister-in-law.

Lars cleared his throat. "I don't think so," he said.

I waited for some sign, for his shoulder to tense again, or for him to jiggle his foot.

My brother jumped in to outline the agenda for the memorial. "Dad's service starts at noon," he said and began to divvy up the chores. I shot him a look of gratitude.

That night in our room with the blackout drapes drawn, tucked under a burnt orange comforter, I turned to Lars in the dark, "Are you sure you don't want to see your family while we're here?"

"I'm sure. There's no point."

He turned away. I followed him across the king-size bed and put my arm around his belly, pulling us into a spoon shape. Minutes later, a faint snore, and no more was said.

CHAPTER 7
MANHATTAN

My father's memorial service was held in the music room at the Actor's Fund Home. My brother gave a tribute. Several of Dad's students who had had successful acting careers lauded his energy and dedication. A pianist played songs from "Damn Yankees" and "Most Happy Fella." We sang along to "Ya Gotta Have Heart," one of Dad's favorites.

He used to belt out that song in the mornings while he was shaving. It made me smile and cry at the same moment. Lars squeezed my hand, but he didn't sing.

Dad had given precise instructions that his cremains be scattered in the Hudson River at a point directly across from his former apartment building in Washington Heights. Tim found a spot on the New Jersey side in Palisades Park that matched my father's instructions. My brother had dumped the ashes in the river the night before.

After the celebration ended, we drove there so he could show us the spot. We piled out of our cars and walked for half a mile, and then crowded onto a bench by the Hudson River admiring the Manhattan skyline.

My sister insisted she could see Dad's ten-story building across the river.

"How can you possibly tell?" I challenged Tess.

For fuck's sake, all the buildings look alike, I wanted to say.

I was cranky in a way you can only be cranky when you're overflowing with unspoken grief, so irritated that suddenly the hairs on the back of my arms stood up.

"That's not Dad's building," I insisted.

Lars had his arm around me. He clenched my shoulder as if to silently say, "Hey now, lighten up."

It infuriated me.

Then Tim jumped in, metaphorically separating Tess and me.

"Whatever it is, Dad is happy. I put his ashes exactly where he asked me to."

I stood up and paced behind the bench. I pictured my father's grainy remains swirling in the uncertain currents of the Hudson River. It was so *him*, so outrageously dramatic.

Lars fit in by keeping quiet and being helpful. He had endeared himself to Tess at the memorial service by helping to set up the flower arrangements and guest book, fussing with the sound system, and setting up the microphone.

Now, he turned to her. "Whether or not it's his building, at least it overlooks the river. He probably used to look out of his window right at this spot where we're sitting."

Okay, I thought. *He's placating her. He's no dummy.*

On the way back to the car, Lars played some Zydeco music on his iPhone, and we positively bounced into the parking lot keeping time to the rhythm. My sister had said how much she loved dancing. Lars spontaneously took her in his arms and began waltzing her around the hot asphalt. He was such a great leader that she managed to follow him, although the look on her face was just short of panic. After a minute, he released her, grasped her hand, and lifted it to his lips for a courtly kiss.

She blushed, overcome by his over-the-top gallantry.

Afterward, Tim drove us to the city for a celebratory dinner at Lattanzi Cucina Italiana, Dad's favorite restaurant in the theater district. The waiters, attired in tuxedos, stood at attention against the exposed brick walls. There were red velvet curtains, crystal chandeliers, crisp white tablecloths, and mahogany chairs with cushy upholstered seats. It was the kind of overdone opulence my father loved.

We toasted to Dad as we munched on fried artichoke hearts and heaped giant mounds of pasta on our plates, all served family style.

"Lucky Boy" was memorable. Tom Hanks played the lead. We had orchestra seats about halfway back and I could see saliva spray from his mouth on certain lines as he embodied a brash reporter down on his luck. It was bitingly funny. I passionately wished Nora Ephron were there to see it. I fell in love with Broadway that night. Now I understood why tickets cost more than the elaborate meal we had just eaten. The food was delicious, the play divine.

The next day, New York City sidewalks shimmered with reflected sunlight. The city was jammed with sweaty bodies and suffused with muggy air. It was so humid that I felt as if I was carrying a wet sheet over my head. Lars and I ducked into the lobby of the Time Warner building at Columbus Circle just for the AC. We had spent the late morning at the Frick looking at French furniture and ceramics.

I had forgotten to pack my migraine medication. There I was in ninety-degree heat with ninety-five percent humidity in a strange city with my newish boyfriend to celebrate my father's life while seeing auras.

I leaned into Lars, and his shoulder supported me.

"I have to go somewhere quiet and cool," I said, nausea swamping me in waves.

"Okay," he agreed.

We held hands; I loved that about him. Whenever we were out, he always took my hand. We headed up 59th Street toward a church a few blocks away, Lars half -eading me there. I willed myself forward, silently repeating, *you can make it, you can make it.*

Inside the church, it was dark and cool. At the altar stood a statue of the Blessed Virgin. Lars guided me halfway up the aisle and into a wooden pew. We sat shoulder to shoulder, then without asking, because I didn't have the energy to, I curled my body onto the bench, pulled up my knees, and put my head in his lap.

He stroked my forehead and my damp hair. Like a child, I soaked up comfort, the smooth feel of his palm on my throbbing head, the way he was just there, not talking, not making a big deal out of it, sitting on a hard wooden pew on a broiling Sunday afternoon in a cool, dark church stroking my head. So not what you come to Manhattan to do.

At the end of that half-hour respite, my nausea had passed. My head still throbbed but less than before.

"Thank you," I said. "That helped."

We went back out onto the hot pavement. Something had changed; as if his kindness had plowed a furrow in my heart, I felt softer, more open to whatever might happen next, like bare brown dirt in a warm field. Waiting.

We met my brother and sister-in-law back at Columbus Circle. Tim had gotten us tickets for a jazz concert and dinner at Dizzy's Club Coca-Cola. We settled ourselves at a little café table inside the nightclub and ordered dinner. Alyssa offered me ibuprofen which I gladly accepted. Thankfully, it was dark and air-conditioned.

The Bill Charlap Trio was playing. Our table stood five yards from the stage, directly behind the piano, and as Charlap began to play, "Ages Ago Last Night" I watched his fingers caress the keys and let the music sweep me away. I forgot all about my headache, or why we were even in New York.

Then they played "Autumn in New York" and "The Nearness of You." Ron Carter was sitting in on bass, and I felt as if I were in the presence of a god. Music poured over us like liquid gold. I found Lars's hand under the table, and he squeezed my fingers. It was a moment. In the picture my brother took of us that night, we're grinning like teenagers in front of a red and yellow sign in the nightclub lobby that says "Jazz."

The next morning Tim and Alyssa drove us to the airport. We had sent Dad off in style, Lars had gotten to know my sibs, and I'd seen what a good traveling companion he was, and how deft and diplomatic. I appreciated him for navigating my family's murky waters, even as he'd sidestepped his own.

CHAPTER 8
KEYS

"You seem far away," I said. We sat on my deck drinking iced tea. Lars only nodded. I put my arm around his shoulder, but he shrugged it off.

Ever since we got back from New York, his moods seemed bipolar. Sometimes he seemed cheerful; at other times completely disengaged. I was riveted by the imminent birth of my second grandchild, due in July. His behavior began to wear on me.

We did what passed for arguing, which was me asking "What's wrong? You seem distant, or you seem stressed, or you seem angry..."

Lars stared into space and didn't reply, or he'd say, "I'm coming down with something."

There were no raised voices, nothing to grapple with, no confrontation. Only a vague unease like hazy clouds before a summer thunderstorm.

During the weeks before the delivery, Lars was evicted from his old apartment because the owner wanted to remodel the unit. He mentioned that he was having some issues at work but didn't say what they were. I was tired of prodding him to explain, so I let it go.

I was preoccupied with my thirty-two-year-old daughter Greta and the coming birth, so I didn't fully appreciate, or even register, how stressed he was.

Greta had had a tough go during the birth of her first child three years earlier. Her labor had been induced. Contractions were wildly strong and rolled on and on in a tsunami of pain. I tried to reassure her that the coming birth would be easier. When I awoke each morning at four o'clock filled with worry, I prayed this would turn out to be true.

Amelia was born July thirtieth after easier labor. By early September, she had grown into a chubby, smiley, gregarious baby—already the opposite of three-year-old Zoe, a more sober, self-contained child.

Lars was AWOL; I hadn't seen him in weeks and our phone calls were clipped. He sent me a letter. In it, he said that I was too busy and that he "couldn't get aboard my train." Interesting metaphor, I thought. He was saying I had no sympathy for him—but he seemed not to have any for me, either. Was this his indirect way of saying that he wanted to break up with me?

For several weeks I did nothing. Then I wrote him a card saying I was open to repairing our fractured relationship. I missed him, but I was also exhausted. I wasn't sure whether our love was worth saving, or if either of us had the energy to try.

Out of the blue he called to tell me he'd rented a new apartment, less than a mile from his old one. He sounded genuinely pleased.

"It's nicer than the old one," he said. "Two bedrooms with big closets."

"Two bedrooms. Wow," I said, wondering how he'd managed the magic feat of finding a two-bedroom apartment in a desirable neighborhood.

"Would you like to see it?"

The anticipation in his voice was palpable as if he was inviting me to a sold-out concert.

When I stepped out of my car to the curb, I took in the scene with admiration. The building was white, with two sets of large steps going up in a half circle, and curving railings. It had an air of early twentiethth-century elegance as if it had been built in the run-up to the Great Depression to give an impression of permanence even to folks who rented month to month.

I rang the bell and Lars answered.

"Come in, come in," he said, with customary jollity.

I warmed to the place quickly—the high ceilings, the second bedroom already kitted out as his office, stacks of books and CDs everywhere. I stood back to admire a walk-in closet in the main bedroom. It had wood floors and a leaded glass window above the closet bar, letting in the afternoon light.

"You lucky duck!" I gestured at the window. He beamed.

His massive collection of shirts hung side by side, looking crisp and dry-cleaned with creased sleeves, although I knew he laundered them himself and purchased them at Costco. It was an impressive display.

I complimented him on this larger place with its huge closets and more room for his hundreds of books and CDs which lay scattered on shelves and tabletops, and even stacked in the hallway. I suggested that he buy more bookshelves. Disorder makes me feel confused and dizzy. I can't focus in chaos. But Lars preferred to be surrounded by a fortress of clutter.

At last, it was time to go. He walked me to his new front door. I turned to kiss him, happy that we had finally reconnected. He backed away, then stretched out his hand.

"I'd like my keys back," he said.

He held his hand inches away from me, palm up. I didn't understand at first.

"Your keys?"

"Yes, the keys to my old place," he said.

"Oh," I replied and began digging in my purse.

I drew my lips into a Mona Lisa smile.

"There you go," I said nonchalantly, dropping the keys in his palm.

He took them without comment, or even thanks, then reached in his pocket and removed the green plastic keyring that held the keys to my place.

"Here," he said.

I opened my palm, and he dropped my keys, the cool metal brushing my skin. I put them in my purse as if by getting rid of them quickly I wouldn't understand the implication. It was just simple bookkeeping. Trade his keys for mine.

I let my mind go blank. Lars stood in his open doorway.

"Is this your way of breaking up with me?"

My question hung in the floating dust motes. I glanced at the stacks of books in the hallway behind him, at the wooden coat rack with its curved arms, then looked up at him.

He looked past me as if the Rosetta Stone might be lodged on the tree lawn.

The hum of passing cars whooshed in through his new front door, for which I did not have keys.

"Wow," I said.

I felt like someone had hit my breastbone with a hammer.

I knew instinctively that Lars would not explain or say goodbye or even acknowledge what he was doing. I brushed past him out onto the porch, then into the sunshine and down the stairs in the hot, bright afternoon. I found my car. I unlocked it and got in, fastened my seatbelt, and cranked the ignition.

"Asshole!" I yelled at top volume, as I revved the engine, disengaged the brake, and drove away. I repeated that comforting mantra as I drove home. Twenty minutes later I pulled into my garage.

"That asshole!" I said again as I turned off the motor.

I deserved some explanation, a chance to counter or defend myself, a decent fight for God's sake, not just a pitiful exchange of keys.

I had a prickly sensation behind my eyes and a catch in my throat. What I wanted was a good cry. But it felt more empowering to be angry. Usually, I'm the one who initiates a breakup. But with Lars, despite our miscommunications, his disappearances, my ambivalence, and family diversions, no truly bad behavior had happened.

No one had been unfaithful. No one had lied. Despite our differences, we had similar world views and tastes in music and books. Most of all, I loved *and* liked Lars. He was—up to that moment, at least—a dependable partner and a good friend.

"If someone won't come to the table, you can't make them."

I was sitting across from my employee assistance therapist, Linda, who looked casually elegant—dark hair pulled back in a loose bun, silver hoop earrings, a tailored white shirt with turned-back cuffs under a charcoal gray sweater.

"I honestly don't know why he broke up with me," I said.

It was October, and the sting of Lars's abrupt return of my keys with no explanation had only intensified. At first, I was shocked and outraged, now those emotions had composted down to sadness and profound loneliness. I missed him. The bastard!

Linda nodded sympathetically. Her earrings caught the gleams of the fluorescent office lights. Her bookshelves over-flowed with tomes on psychology, and her office held tasteful lamps with neutral shades, and modern art prints; all standard corporate issue. It was professional, yet cozy. I was grateful for a place to come and expound on my misery.

"You may never know the real reasons," she said. "But that's on Lars, not you."

I nodded back at her, numb with regret.

"But why?" I persisted. "Why won't he explain, or at least give me a chance to ask questions?"

"Maybe he can't," she said. "Some people aren't good at post-mortems; they don't want to repair what's broken."

I picked at a piece of lint on my sweater sleeve considering her words. I stroked the smooth chair arms, thinking about how I couldn't make Lars do anything, least of all explain.

"It leaves me in this weird Limbo," I said.

I remembered confraternity classes when I was a child, having to go every Monday afternoon to Our Lady of the Lake Cath-olic Church where the nun would drill us on our Baltimore Catechism. Limbo stood between heaven and hell. I pictured it as a giant waiting room in a Greyhound bus station full of lost souls waiting to find out where they'd end up. That's how I felt now: a lost soul not knowing what sin I might have committed to make Lars leave me.

"Did you have any idea he planned to break up?" Linda asked.

"He was acting distant," I replied. "I knew he wasn't happy, but I figured we'd have a chance to talk about it."

She had stressed in our sessions that repair was the most vital relationship skill. Everyone screws up, she said. The key is knowing how to forgive, and how to make things right.

I'd always assumed I just didn't know how to be in a relationship, that there was something inherently flawed in my inability to sustain closeness, and that I had "ambivalent attachment" issues, all of which were likely true. But she made me see that was normal—we all have some version of that—it's the human condition. Now, I wouldn't get a chance to put my newfound insights to work. At least not with Lars, damn him.

CHAPTER 9
THE INTERREGNUM

I went dancing at Eagles after a few months. Lars looked past me when I walked towards him as if he didn't know me. I thought to myself, *Wow, dude, really?!*

I was wearing tight black pants and a creme silk top, too tight to be a tunic, too long for a blouse; it was flirty without crossing the line into desperation. I fingered my necklace of rhinestone beads like a rosary as I passed him, rubbing my fingers against the cool glass.

Another guy I'd danced with before came up behind me and tapped me on the shoulder. As we swayed and spun to the rhythm of the accordion, I gave in to happiness. Zydeco did that for me. It was better than Ativan, or pot, or even a good glass of Sauvignon Blanc.

Later in the evening, Lars approached my table and extended his hand.

"Would you care to dance?"

I raised an eyebrow. *You're just going to pretend you never broke up with me? That what happened doesn't matter?* But I said nothing. I let him lead me out on the floor. His palm felt warm against my spine, and he guided me firmly into a waltz, which he led flawlessly—just the right amount of pressure on my palm and back with the right distance between us. I felt guided and taken care of. A hiccup of sadness for what could have been burbled up my chest.

I'd called and emailed him several times during September and October with no response. As Linda observed, he just didn't want to come to the table. My anger had softened but I was still curious. Why had he ditched me?

I looked up at him. He met my gaze and then looked away.

"How have you been?" I inquired. "I've been worried. I wasn't sure what happened to you. I wondered, is he dead in a ditch? Kidnapped by aliens?"

Lars didn't crack a smile, not so much as an eye roll or a shrug. He was solid as a piece of granite, albeit one that was a fabulous dancer.

"Seriously, Lars, why haven't you returned my calls?"

"I was busy," he said, his blue-gray eyes darkening, his shoulders tensing, which I could feel through the crisp cotton of his shirt.

"Okay," I said. "But we were a couple for eight months."

I was counting from the first time he had told me he loved me, last February, sitting on my couch, not from the first time we had sex, the evening of the day my father had died. Eight months is a good amount of time, I thought. *You owe me an explanation.*

But Lars didn't see it that way.

A pattern developed. I'd see him on Friday nights at Eagles. Sometimes we'd talk before the dance. Our conversations focused on the book he was reading because invariably he was reading while waiting for the music to begin. It was usually something very esoteric or nerdy: *Why We Sleep,* or *Thermodynamics,* or

Thucydides on the Peloponnesian Wars. I'd gently poke fun at him or ask questions if I was interested in the topic. Often, we'd dance a few dances; then it might be weeks before we'd talk or dance again.

As time passed, I grew less obsessed with the mystery, and began to accept the reality: Lars wasn't coming back. He didn't owe me a thing, no matter what I thought I deserved, or how much I longed to know why.

※

One night when Lars and I were waltzing I fell into a hypnotic reverie, a dream state. I remember as a kid being fascinated by a couple who lived on our street in a neat little white bungalow with red shutters, Ed and his wife Nids, whose real name was Margaret. They lived four doors up the street from us. Ed was a plumber, and Nids a housewife. She used to vacuum their carpet every day, while my mother only vacuumed once a week.

Nids had dyed black hair and wore red lipstick and black mascara. She smoked Pall Malls, which we used to steal from her purse. Her figure was a classic Marilyn Monroe-style hourglass with a narrow waist. She often wore black patent leather belts that cinched dresses with full skirts. Ed wore beige work clothes, matching pants, and shirts, with his name embroidered on the shirt pocket, and came home every afternoon at four o'clock, sharp, with a toolbox he'd take out of his station wagon and stash in their back entry.

When he came home, they always kissed. Sometimes we'd be in the kitchen, their daughter Maureen and me, bugging Nids for cookies or a popsicle. But when Ed came in the room, Nid's face lit up like a movie star, and he'd grab her waist and pull her towards him in front of the sink, wrapping his arms around her, tugging. I couldn't stop staring. They'd kiss, and their lips would mesh, a little deeper, lasting a little longer, not like the hunt and peck that passed for kissing at my house.

One time, Maureen told me she went down to the basement looking for something. Ed and Nids had fallen asleep on the couch in their rec room, and Ed's hand was cupped under Nid's right breast, her head on his shoulder, his thrown back against the couch. To me, that seemed like something out of a risqué foreign movie. Nobody's parents fell asleep on the rec room couch and stayed there all night. Ed and Nids were my romantic ideal, even with all that vacuuming. There was a lot of love in that house, and it wasn't the platonic kind.

When Lars put his hand on the small of my back as if he was holding a Ming vase, as if I might shatter if he handled me too roughly, it made me think of Ed and Nids. How Ed always had a half grin on his face, his soft voice husky; how Nids always seemed upbeat about vacuuming. Looking back, they were one of the few happy couples I knew.

I let Lars sweep me over the dance floor, holding me in that competent solid way of his. In those moments, it was as if we'd never broken up. We were still moving together, in rhythm; he was still holding me.

Then I remembered that during lovemaking Lars would touch me the same way, carefully, as if he was in Biology class, looking at me through a microscope, examining me, then moving me into position for a closer look. Lars is a scientist, I thought, an explorer. He had a way of investigating my body that was slow, thorough, as if studying every part in an orderly sequence, working his way from my head and lips to my neck, then to my breasts, my belly, and then pulling my legs apart and positioning himself squarely at my body's opening, his lips and tongue exploring with the same precision as if he was moving me around the dance floor. He was methodical, in sex, in dance, in life.

I thought those memories would make me sad, but they didn't. He was still holding me, still guiding me, still moving me to the music. True, we were no longer a couple—I was even dating another of my dance partners by this time—but somehow Lars and I were still connected.

I managed to keep it light with him. "What are you reading?" or "How are your parents doing?" rather than asking what I wanted to know: "Why did you break up with me?"

I tried to accept that I'd probably never find out, but that didn't stop me from wanting to know. I focused on enjoying Lars in the moment, his hand on my back, his way of guiding me across the dance floor, and how he always walked me back to my chair after we danced.

I didn't know then what I would learn later: that when the time came, those years of becoming friends would make us better partners, that our separation mysteriously created a new, stronger foundation. Perhaps we needed to learn what could drive us apart so that later we'd be prepared. At last, we would discover how much it felt like we were starving during our time out, and how much desire mattered.

When anyone asks about our origin story, we recount our sudden breakup, but we tell it differently.

"You mean our interregnum?" That's how Lars refers to the breakup. As if we were deposed monarchs.

"I was in a bad frame of mind," he'll say, and then recount how his landlord had just evicted him to remodel the apartment, and how his boss was being an abusive jerk, although that's not the way Lars would phrase it.

"Honey, it was more than that," I'll say. "You were feeling as if I wasn't paying enough attention to you."

Then he'll demur. "Not exactly," he'll say.

"Yes, exactly," I'll say. "Greta was about to give birth. I was worried because her first labor was so difficult. I wasn't focused on you."

I'll remind him about the afternoon when he asked for his keys. He'll nod but say nothing. I'll remind him of the goodbye note I wrote to him acknowledging our breakup, saying the words he wouldn't or couldn't say, and thanking him for our time together.

Then, I'll say, "Remember the time I apologized to you?" By that point, four years had passed since the afternoon Lars had left me abruptly.

We were on the dance floor at Eagles one night when something came over me, something I urgently needed to say. I looked up at him.

"Lars, before you broke up with me, I was very happy."

He reared back and looked down at me.

"But I wasn't," he said.

"I know that now," I said.

I went on, "I want to sincerely apologize for whatever it was that I said or did to make you unhappy."

It had only taken the years apart, and another disastrous breakup, to make me believe that Lars was by far the best applicant for the job of being my partner. Enough time for me to grow softer, to be more vulnerable, to admit that I was also at fault.

"I'm sorry," I had said, looking straight into Lars's eyes.

We kept on dancing. Nothing more was said that night, but something had shifted.

PART II
SECOND CHANCES

CHAPTER 10
A FISH WITHOUT A BICYCLE

I shuffled downstairs. Hearing my knock, my neighbor Chloe peered through the peephole and unlocked the door.

"Hey," I said. "Are you busy? I need a friend..."

My hair was a mess. I peered at her with red-rimmed eyes. I looked as awful as I felt.

I'd spent the morning in flannel PJs, lying on my couch watching old Downton Abbey episodes to distract myself. I'd be okay and then mysteriously crying. For what?

"Come in, come in," she said and whisked me through the door, locking it behind me.

Chloe was twenty-five years younger than me, attractive, slim, and neurotic as hell. She worked ungodly hours in a hospital intensive care unit as a nurse and made gobs of money. Every day there were piles of Amazon boxes outside her door—clothes, toys for her cats, immersion blenders, new handbags. Whatever. She had admitted she had a problem.

I liked her even more for it.

She gestured to the couch. I snuggled in.

Two years after Lars dumped me, I began dating another one of my dance partners. We had dated for more than a year with minor disagreements, and I thought things were going well. Then we took a five-week trip to Europe, and I discovered I was mistaken.

I had yelled at him on a street corner in Palma, Mallorca for treating me like an unpaid tour guide. We'd been traveling for four weeks by then and my patience was wearing thin.

"Read the fucking itinerary," I seethed between clenched teeth after Saeed asked me for the umpteenth time why we were visiting the art museum in Palma on a Tuesday morning.

He stared at me dumbstruck.

"I'm not your secretary," I hissed to underline the point.

He was a seventy-five-year-old former businessman who had emigrated from Dubai and promoted the fiction that he was six years younger than his actual age, which should have been a clue that he suffered from an inflated ego. Also, when he drove the wrong way in a parking garage, blocking all the incoming cars, I suspected he had cognitive issues.

I apologized profusely within a few hours, admitting that I'd crossed a line. He sulked for the rest of the trip. Then, after we returned home, I found myself on a merry-go-round. One minute he would charm me into giving our relationship a second chance, the next he'd be ranting at me about what a disappointment I was.

Saeed gave me the boot on Thanksgiving Day along with a tongue-lashing that exceeded my outburst by a factor of ten. Unlike Lars, who said nothing before breaking up with me, this guy had overshared. I was still recovering.

"Some of the horrible things he said held a grain of truth," I admitted to Chloe. "I had to take a second look at how I do relationships."

What I didn't admit was that on top of the hideous breakup, my novel had been rejected by an agent I had hoped would represent me. I had put heart and soul into the last round of revisions, and when the agent's assistant asked to see the entire manuscript, I was elated. So, when they turned it down, I was crushed.

The last two years of effort—the countless drafts, the expensive sessions with a developmental editor, the exchange of pages with fellow writers—all seemed pointless, and even a little grandiose. Who did I think I was, anyway?

I told myself not to take it personally. I gave myself pep talks about getting my butt back in the chair. I called up writer friends who commiserated and assured me that brighter days lay ahead. Nothing worked. That's when I gave in to the couch.

We talked about the guy Chloe was dating until a few weeks ago. He had seemed so promising. Dinners out. Flowers. Concerts. Even a few weekend trips. Then he dropped the bombshell that he had decided to reunite with an old girlfriend.

"I thought he was the one," she said, reaching for a Kleenex. She had a box tucked into the corner of her leather couch.

"What a jerk!" I felt sorry for her, I really did.

Then we discussed the merits of various anti-depressants and I confessed that I'd recently had to switch back to my old prescription of long-acting Wellbutrin.

"It takes a while to build up in your bloodstream," she observed.

"No joke," I said. "Please pass the Kleenex."

I had to ride it out while I waited for the new/old pills to arrive and for the drug, my depleted dopamine, and my weepy self to get back in sync.

I sensed that Chloe and I were winding down.

"Thanks for listening," I said, rising to leave.

"I'm glad you dropped by," she said.

I trudged back upstairs.

Out my window, I looked down at the tops of the sycamore trees along Lakeshore Avenue, a row of tile rooves, red brick chimneys, and backyards full of electric pink bougainvillea draped elegantly over fences. The cross street wended its way to Crocker Highlands, an Oakland neighborhood of mansions, some ivy-covered with leaded glass windows.

I've always been a limpet, attaching myself to the edges of upper-crust life, clinging to fading gentility, the leftovers from my grandmother's table. I liked trees, open space, peace, and order. So, I perched near the rich or almost rich. I was "wealth adjacent," having had the good sense to buy my unit right after the crash of 2008.

I felt better. I made a sandwich. Maybe all was not lost, after all.

The Wellbutrin kicked in. I got back to work at the office I shared with a group of fellow writers in San Francisco, slogging away on revising my novel for the third time, trusting that it would all be worth it.

At day's end, I hiked down 2nd Street dragging my computer bag, dodging twenty-somethings in brightly colored Vans and skinny jeans. Most of them looked too young to deliver papers or mow lawns, let alone write code or work on perfecting the human/machine interface. I imagined they made gazillions, had six roommates, spent two weeks a year in Paris, and were staggering under mountains of student debt.

I knew they only looked so fresh-faced to me because I was old, yet I persisted in thinking of them as interlopers in the city, while I was a seasoned pro.

A few blocks over on New Montgomery Street there's a vintage condo building that used to house the old phone company headquarters. I worked there for ten years editing the company magazine, as a comparative youngster in my forties, raising two kids, living paycheck to paycheck, and commuting from Walnut Creek. I spent hours bent over my desk, toiling away under deadline, a whiteboard on the wall with a list of stories for the current issue scratched out in washable marker. In hindsight, it was a dream job.

But back then, it was hellfire and brimstone with occasional flashes of humor. The colleague who used to remind me "We are just lackeys of the ruling classes," or the production manager who would say, sotto voce, "Butts up kneeling," every time one of the vice presidents came to visit our floor.

We had some laughs while I hauled myself up by the boot-straps, got out of debt, contributed to my 401K, and took a buyout when I had the chance. Now, I bowed to the old granite building, acknowledging that I was able to write a novel only because I worked my privileged butt off in corporate jobs for thirty years, and had a pension and savings.

I parted the young folks like Moses at the Red Sea, a lone woman in jeans with a streak of silver in her hair, immersed in her third act, walking toward the BART station.

I passed the guy with a German Shepherd sitting by the BART staircase holding a cardboard sign that read "I'm hungry, and so is my dog." I wanted to cry.

Back in the day, I ran down the steps like everyone else, rushed through the fare gate and down the escalator, so I wouldn't be late to pick up my kids, get dinner on the table, supervise homework, and get them to bed. Now, I took my time, held the handrail, and watched my step.

I didn't even have a cat to rush home for anymore. Saffron had crossed the Rainbow Bridge several months before.

When I disembarked in Oakland, I walked up 20th Street toward Lake Merritt, dawdling in front of Starbucks, tempted by the thought of a Chai latte, decided against it, and then did some window shopping at Janko's Jewelers.

I used to get my watch batteries replaced at Janko's and linger at the glass counters, finding mixed metal earrings I liked on the display stands. Right before I retired in 2015, I treated myself to a pearl pendant on a gold chain.

A bell chimed when I pushed open the glass door, and one of the owners welcomed me in, greeting me by name.

"I haven't seen you in two years.

"Yeah, I retired. I'm working in the city now."

"Doing what?

"Writing full time."

Margo raised a sculpted eyebrow.

"Good for you," she said. "So, what can I help you with?"

"Just browsing," I said, looking down at a display of rings on a velvet tray.

A ring with a luminous pearl set with diamond chips on each side caught my eye. My grandmother Pearl used to let us watch daytime soap operas, eat Milky Ways, and stay up to watch the late movie, so I associate all that spoiling with pearls. Plus, my parents who expected a son as their firstborn and found they needed a name for a daughter instead, named me after my grandmothers: Eleanor for Mom's mom, and Pearl for Dad's mom.

Both of us looked lovingly at the tray of rings. Margo followed my gaze.

"Would you like to see one?"

I pointed through the glass. "The pearl and diamond one, third in from the left," I said.

She lifted it out and held it up to the light. I was tantalized by its sparkle.

"Try it on," she urged.

I slipped it on my right-hand ring finger. It fit perfectly.

"How much?" I inquired, knowing it was going to be more than I could afford.

She quoted me a less than jaw-dropping but still hefty price, then reminded me I could put it on layaway.

"It's more likely I'm going to be killed by a terrorist than have a man buy me this ring," I mused. "It's gorgeous. I love it. My seventieth birthday is coming up in six months. I could buy this ring and get engaged to myself. I'll amortize it over the time I own it and love it. If I live to be 95, it will only cost me a few bucks a month!"

Less than I'd spend on one latte! It seemed a reasonable price to pay for the sparkle.

"You're a customer of long-standing," Margo said. "I'll knock two hundred off the price, and you have six months to pay."

That sealed the deal. I handed her my credit card for the down payment.

Eleanor Pearl Vincent, will you marry me?

I chuckled. She smiled. We were both delighted. I took off the ring and she polished it with a soft cloth until it gleamed, then wrote my name on a little Manilla envelope, popped the ring inside, and handed back my card.

What was that feminist saying from the 1970s? "A woman without a man is like a fish without a bicycle."

I floated out of the store and walked home on Grand Avenue along the edge of Lake Merritt swimming happily upstream.

CHAPTER 11
LARS TO THE RESCUE

One early December evening, I set out for home after a long day in San Francisco. It was my second week of butt-back-in-the-chair. I'd revised a couple of novel chapters and commiserated over lunch with my writing pals. On top of that, I planned to stop at Janko's Jewelers and make a payment on my ring. I'd finally accepted that I'd be single for the rest of my life and that seemed if not peachy, at least manageable.

When I arrived home that Friday, I unlocked my door, threw down my purse and computer bag, switched on the PBS News Hour, poured a half glass of Sauvignon Blanc, and settled back on my couch cushions. I was in a TGIF frame of mind.

Suddenly the oblong black eye of my iPhone flashed to life. Perhaps a text from a friend? A Facebook notification? Breaking news from my *New York Times* app?

I purchased my first iPhone so that I could text my daughter Greta. Texting on my flip phone was ridiculously difficult. Once I had the phone, an expensive piece of technology one rarely uses to *talk* to anyone, I found I could text to my heart's content and Greta would respond. Phone tag was a thing of the past.

I picked up the phone to find a reminder: there was a new version of IOS waiting to be downloaded. I knew better than to fall into that trap. Those downloads can take for-fricking-ever. I set the phone down, took another sip of wine, and refocused my attention on Judy Woodruff.

I loved my iPhone's bright icons—blue, fuchsia, Kelly green, and basic black. I adored the satisfying click it made when I tapped. I double loved my phone camera. Photo after photo for me to edit, enhance, or delete, photos I could snap on the spur of the moment and post in an instant. Photos I saved for eons right there on the screen to share with my older granddaughter Zoe—it kept her happy in restaurants while we were waiting for our French Fries.

Bit by enticing bit, I had grown ever more dependent on my iPhone. My calendar, my maps, my addresses and phone numbers, my glorious photos—everything of vital importance lived inside that shiny black screen with its bright icons.

So, when I went to bed that night, I plugged in the phone and permitted it to install the new operating system.

The next morning when I woke up, I snuggled deeper under the duvet and began debating breakfast offerings. I reached for my phone on the bedside table, but the table was bare. I panicked. Then I remembered. I'd started the new IOS download.

I padded into the living room to check on the phone. The battery icon said one hundred percent. I composed a text for Greta and hit send. There was a pause, and the screen went black. Black!

I tried again. Again, the phone crashed. Again, I restarted it and hit the blue weather icon with the yellow sun and white cloud. Boom. Black screen. My heart raced. I felt dizzy and mildly nauseous. My digital life flashed before my eyes. Then I thought of Lars.

I composed a text. *Hey Lars—my iPhone crashes whenever I hit an icon. What to do?*

I hit send. I felt as if I was in a dropping elevator as the phone went black again. My breath came in shallow gulps and the muscles in the back of my neck tensed. My whole life existed inside this rectangle!

Desperate, I pulled up Lars's number in my contacts and ran to my cordless phone, now an antique. My call went to voice mail, and I blurted out a few strangled words.

A few minutes later, I got a text from Lars. *What's up? I got a missed call from you.*

I texted back. *SOS, iPhone crash. Please help!*

By a miracle, I pressed the arrow key and the text box turned blue. It had gone out.

The phone crashed again. I turned it on again.

Incoming text from Lars, *I'm on my way over.*

I took a deep belly breath and set the phone down. If anyone could figure out why it was behaving so strangely, it would be Lars. No technology glitch or crash phased him. With years of experience, he had the confidence to know he—or Apple support—could fix everything.

Technology mystified me. I would no more know how to troubleshoot my phone than how to change the oil in my car. And I was just about as interested. Which is to say, not at all.

Five years had passed since that November night at Eagles when Lars asked me to dance. Six months after our breakup we started over as dance partners and friends, and in the last year, we'd grown closer. Sometimes, I'd reach out just to chat, or send a supportive text as he dealt with his parents' final illnesses and their deaths. Whenever a computer question plagued me, I consulted Lars.

When the doorbell chimed, I flew to answer it. Lars was wearing his yellow Nepalese wool scarf, his customary brushed felt fedora, and a black wool jacket. He might as well have worn a cape, and tights, and sported a giant red S on his chest.

"My hero," I gushed. "Please come in."

"Have you tried turning it off and on?"

I felt as if we were in an episode of the British comedy "The IT Crowd," it was such a classic tech support question.

"Of course," I said. "But it's doing a very good job of that all on its own."

I hung his jacket in the closet and stashed his hat and scarf on the desk by the door.

"I'm making breakfast. Are you hungry?"

"Maybe later," Lars said. He extended his hand for the iPhone.

I handed it over like a naughty child I was sending to a time-out. Lars took it and headed into my office where he had often fixed laptop issues or done emergency backups for me.

Moments later, I heard him describing the problem to an Apple support technician.

I was happy to let him handle the technology while I dealt with something that made me feel comforted: preparing a hearty breakfast.

Light flooded the kitchen, licking the edges of the living room carpet. I could hear my neighbor banging the lid of her washer, starting a new load, then silence as she transferred clothes to the dryer. Her laundry room was adjacent to my living room wall, and our midcentury building had no soundproofing When the dryer began to hum, she yelled something to one of her kids. It felt so quintessentially Saturday morning that I didn't mind the noise; it felt as comforting as a cup of hot chocolate.

I busied myself making pancake batter—a quarter cup of oil, an egg, the buttermilk and flour mix, then the perfume of a teaspoon of vanilla and some cinnamon. I mixed gently with a wooden spoon, feeling sunlight splash over my shoulders, warming my hands.

By the time Lars finished his call, breakfast would be ready. His voice rose and fell in the office. This too was reassuring. He was so calm. He was figuring out why my phone had crashed. Soon, it would be fixed.

A stack of bacon sat between two paper towels, and the smell of bacon grease permeated the kitchen. Pancakes and bacon reminded me of cold winter mornings in Pennsylvania when the warmth of the stove melted the frost forming on the inside of the kitchen windows.

Oakland winters consisted of fog and rain, not snow and ice. But the feeling of coziness was the same—pancakes and syrup made everything feel safer, more predictable.

Now, the oven warmth mingled with the sunshine. My cheeks felt flushed. The bacon grease and the frying pancakes mingled into a heavenly aroma.

After 20 minutes of surfing the Apple website, and talking with the technician, Lars pinpointed the problem. There was a bug in the new version of IOS I'd downloaded the night before. To fix it, we'd have to delete and reload all my apps. When he told me, I groaned.

"I can't face it without pancakes," I said. "C'mon, let's eat."

I carried our plates to the table.

"It's been a while for pancakes," Lars said. "Looks delicious."

"Thank you so much for saving the day," I said. "Breakfast is the least I can do."

Two hours later, the phone was fixed, we'd deleted and reinstalled my apps, and Lars had backed up the phone and my laptop. He had given up his Saturday morning to rescue me. I was beyond grateful. I enjoyed his company. I'd fed him breakfast. It felt like old times, and I began to wonder why on earth we had ever broken up in the first place.

"Was it all just a crazy misunderstanding?"

I straightened up from loading the last plate in the dishwasher and looked at him.

"What?"

"Our breakup. What were we thinking?"

He laughed. "I'm not sure I remember."

Then he took me in his arms and danced me around the kitchen. I knew better than to expect a deep discussion about a sensitive topic: that was not Lars's style. So, I relaxed into his arms, enjoying the moment.

CHAPTER 12
STRAWBERRY PIE

Dwarfed by a matte black construction the size of two Ikea bookshelves, Lars and I gazed at *Mirror Image I, 1969*. We were at the San Jose Museum of Art, entranced by Louise Nevelson's sculptures. Nevelson had long been one of my heroes, an exemplar of creative power, and I was excited to share her work with my beloved.

The piece is built from dozens of wood scraps stacked inside crates, the kind of monumental work that made Nevelson famous, that blurs the line between sculpture and painting. Soaked in black paint so dense it conjured the absence rather than the presence of color, the space between objects punctuated each shape with shadows. My brain shifted from deep to shallow and back, a dizzying sensation.

"Look at the way the shapes repeat from top to bottom and side to side," I said.

Lars inclined his head, considering. He was drawn to the squares and rectangles; I loved the wavy, irregular shapes.

I reached for his hand, and we interlaced our fingers. His thumb pad was fleshy, and his palm warmed mine. It was the opposite of the afternoon five years before when he had dropped his cold keys in my hand and asked for his in return. Now that he had circled back, I basked in his warmth, and I told myself we would find a way to make it work.

Lars had a Kiwanis event to attend in San Jose, and I was a passionate devotee of Nevelson's art. I suggested we combine the two on a January afternoon in 2018.

Lars was reverent about art. He collected books by the hundreds and owned dozens that explored color theory or aesthetics. In this, we converged, never happier than in a museum or gallery, at a concert or a play.

I moved across the gallery, drawn to a photo of Nevelson attired in one of her iconic costumes—a richly patterned silk vest with Chinese dragons, her signature chunky jewelry, and a black felt cap. A double layer of mink eyelashes framed her deep-set eyes. Her career was hard-won during the 1940s and '50s when, as a woman who made massive sculptures, she was relegated to the margins. She had been poor, rejected, and ignored.

So, the mink eyelashes and colorful silk were an understandable self-aggrandizement once she finally found success.

I had interviewed Nevelson when I was in my mid-twenties, a graduate student in the Journalism school at the University of Minnesota. I was working as a reporter at *The Minnesota Daily*. My beat was women's issues and culture. Nevelson was the perfect amalgam of the two—a feminist icon who broke boundaries and changed the game for women who followed.

We sat in her Minneapolis hotel suite, me, a green twenty-five-year-old with a notebook on my knee, a new mother trying to balance writing with caregiving. Nevelson, seventy-four, was alternately imperious and affectionate as we spoke. I was overawed by her, magnetized by her aphorisms.

She was about to launch an exhibit at the Walker Art Center in the fall of 1973. Art critics from the major local newspapers were alerted, yet she had granted an interview to the university paper to my delight.

After we had talked for half an hour, the PR guy from the Walker came in.

"You have a busy day, Mrs. Nevelson," he said. "Maybe you should wrap it up."

Nevelson winked at me. Then, with elaborate noblesse oblige, she looked over her shoulder and addressed her handler.

"Dear, it's for a student newspaper. Surely, we can have a little more time."

He bowed to her and backed out of the room.

She continued responding to my questions as if the interruption had never happened, then asked me about my work. We talked about the struggle between art and life for women. Nevelson leaned back, jangled her bracelets, and inclining her lined face, fixed me with a piercing gaze.

"For me, people are like ..." I'm not sure what I was expecting. But then she said, "Like you eat strawberry pie. They are not the meat of my life."

I wrote down her words with trembling fingers, taking dictation from a guru. I felt as if she could see how unsure I was, how hard I was trying to be a wife and mother, retracing some thin plot I copied from *Leave it to Beaver*.

I passionately wanted to be a writer. I was terrified of being a writer. I couldn't just leave my baby daughter Maya alone in her crib, disappear to my desk in the attic, and write, could I? With a living myth before me, I felt like a pebble on a vast beach, small, tumbled by the waves. But a pebble with responsibilities.

The thought of Maya's cries pierced my heart. Watching her play in the laundry basket as if it were a magic fairy coach filled me with joy. Leaving my one-year-old was impossible. I could never see my girl as strawberry pie, as merely dessert. She *was* the meat of my life, my true love. But what about my writing?

I looked at Louise Nevelson, then at the scribbled words on the pages of my notebook.

I couldn't imagine being as single-minded and necessarily selfish. She had divorced her rich husband and left her baby son with her mother. She had been poor and scorned for her choices. She told me she had been so hungry she would sometimes sleep with a man just to get a hot meal. But her art was her *real* food.

At last, I closed my notebook, we shook hands and went our separate ways. Yet even now, here in a museum gallery, with Lars by my side, I could hear her gravelly voice saying, "For me, people are like"—she paused and waved her hands as if swatting away an insect—"they are like you eat strawberry pie. They are not the meat of my life."

I stood in front of Nevelson's photo, rooted to the spot, arguing with her. Had I chosen wisely? I had not put the people I loved in second place and elevated my creative life above all else. With two kids by two different men, two divorces, and the work it took to support us, I just kept on marching. But I also kept writing.

In my mind, I saw that young woman with a notebook on her knee. *Thank God she didn't know what awaited her*, I thought, that baby who eighteen years later would fall from a horse she was riding bareback and die. Who could have imagined that the book I'd been waiting years to write would be about losing the girl who could never be strawberry pie?

After Maya died and my younger daughter Greta left home for college, I finally pivoted and made writing central. But there had been those three decades before, the long slog of childrearing and breadwinning, the many times writing took a backseat.

In 2018 I was about to turn seventy, a little younger than Nevelson had been when I interviewed her, still trying to find a workable balance.

Later, I told Lars what Nevelson had said about strawberry pie.

"Relationships were optional for her, like dessert, not where she found true nourishment," I explained.

He nodded but remained silent, his eyebrows furled. His silences unnerved me, but I knew he'd clam up if I inquired. I imagined that he thought Nevelson was right, that her dictum made perfect sense. Possibly not for the same reasons, though.

I picked up the exhibit catalog in the museum gift store. In it, there was a signature Nevelson aphorism. I read it aloud.

"You see, you can buy the whole world and you are empty, but when you create the whole world, you are full."

"I can't afford the whole world," Lars joked. "Who would want to buy it, anyway?"

He put his arm around my shoulders and ushered me into the crisp January night. I leaned in. He smelled like soap and his favorite body oil, Night Rain, and his wool coat scratched my cheek. He had glossed over her point. Nevelson was talking about the primacy of creative work, about the meat of her life. Lars focused on the empty part, the part about buying the world.

Would I be like strawberry pie to Lars? I wondered. *And what would he be to me?*

He drove us to the Kiwanis dinner, navigating six lanes of freeway traffic as if he were buttering a slice of bread. He shimmied the car between two huge SUVs at the Hyatt Regency and made it look easy.

Navigating life in the real world was his superpower. Rush hour traffic, too small parking spaces, and misbehaving computers, which he handled like a digital lion tamer, never fazed him. He opened the car door for me, took my hand, and walked me across the parking lot. We went into a too-bright lobby, and he ushered me to the bar.

He is an expert at cocktail chatter. He does it gaily, gliding on the surface. I abhor it. My idea of hell is a party where I don't know anyone. But there he was, tall and distinguished in a suit jacket and tie. So solid. I took a deep breath and walked into a huge ballroom by his side.

At dinner, we sat with six strangers at a round table. I patted the tablecloth's starchy surface, then fingered the napkin in my lap, leaning in to catch the conversation. The words were like hummingbirds, buzzing and hovering over the table.

"We went to Medellin. There's a big Kiwanis presence there, ten clubs."

"Did you work on the Polio eradication project?"

Lars listened intently. He asked intelligent questions. I was interested in the Columbian city, which seemed foreign and exotic, but within moments I was deathly bored. I retraced my steps through the gallery. I saw Nevelson's face in my mind, wondering how her kind of artistic freedom might have changed me.

I sipped my wine, a beautiful rosé, catching the light as I swirled my glass. *I should try harder to engage,* I told myself. But they were talking about irrigation canals and Polio clinics. I let my affable beloved carry the conversation. I laughed at appropriate moments and watched Lars be his Kiwanis self, the man who does good works. It was one of the qualities that made me love him. He wanted to help. Acts of service were his love language.

A museum exhibit combined with a dinner for one of the largest volunteer organizations in the world was an odd juxtaposition. Yet it meshed the things we loved.

That outing with its bits and bobs, its art and commerce, its introspection and cocktail chit-chat, cemented our reconciliation. In all the ways I was a bit dented, Lars was whole, and vice versa.

We both loved to disappear into a good book, a great movie, or a museum gallery, although our interpretations of what we saw or read were wildly different. Nevelson's dictum worked in opposite ways for us. I wanted the main course *and* the dessert, people I love encircling me. Lars preferred people to be like appetizers—intriguing but fleeting.

I have a photo of us at the Kiwanis dinner that night. We're toasting with stemmed glasses of wine, grinning like fools, about to test the boundary between necessary selfishness and love.

CHAPTER 13
COLLISION

When we returned to each other, our bodies moved with such velocity it was as if we had pushed a parked car down a hill, ran to catch it, snatched open the doors and jumped into the back seat, and began ripping off each other's clothes as the car raced down the hill.

A few weeks after our museum visit, Lars invited me to visit his apartment and left the door unlocked because he wanted to take a nap. When I arrived, I stole into his room, removed my shoes, and climbed in next to him dressed in jeans and a sweater. When I touched his cheek, his eyes fluttered open and he smiled.

"Hello, gorgeous," he said.

"Hey, handsome," I replied.

We were like Amish teenagers tied together fully clothed for a session of "bundling," a custom that precedes marriage and is meant to kindle the fires of passion. The aim is to be frustrated on purpose.

Lars and I rubbed noses. Then we kissed luxuriously and rounded the bases, stopping before we reached home plate, ravenous with desire.

I emerged from his bed with scratch marks across my lower back and a bite on my neck, fully satisfied. We didn't do the deed. We both needed more time to absorb what was happening. Our speeding car was not exactly a little red Corvette!

As I gathered my purse to head back to my house, he asked me to wait.

I already had a hand on the front door, anticipating a hot bath and the comforts of my own sweet home.

He emerged from his office with a gift bag stuffed with tissue paper and held it out to me as if it were a Valentine.

"Open it," he said.

I fished out two silver keys as well as a black plastic fob, which I assumed was a key ring, from the mound of tissue. Lars said these were the keys to the apartment. He proceeded to demonstrate how to lock and unlock the front door, which was a little touchy. I needed him to tutor me as I fumbled with the keys.

I was so focused on learning the quirks of the locks that I didn't question what Lars intended with this little surprise.

"I have to go," I said. "Thanks for the keys."

He gave me a puzzled look, then kissed the top of my head. Like a child, eager for her next adventure, I waltzed out of his front door without a second thought.

Later, when I phoned to let him know I was safely home, he blurted, "The black fob is the key to my car."

"Wait," I said. "You mean to your *new* car?"

"Yes."

"*What?* You gave me the key to your car?"

I was incredulous. "Why?" That seemed like the next logical question.

"Because I'm all in," he responded after a pause.

"Please give me some context," I begged. "I don't get it."

He patiently explained that giving me the keys to his house and car was the equivalent of a solemn promise that he would never leave me. That's what he meant by "all in." I was touched but still mystified.

I'd never had a car with keyless entry. The black fob was a mysterious piece of black plastic to me, nothing more. I had completely missed the significance of the keys.

Then, Lars explained that he had been crushed by my casual response to this very important gift.

"I'm so glad you told me," I said. "I had no way of knowing what it meant."

It was terrifying for me to confront the different ways we interpreted the simplest gestures. This misunderstanding broke over my head in waves. I felt like I'd been so eager to get home that I hadn't taken the time to ask Lars what he had intended.

"Thank you," I said. "I'm honored to have your keys."

After we hung up, I wondered if it would ever be possible for me to understand Lars, or to accurately translate his actions. He was so subtle. I felt sad that I had missed his meaning.

At first, I thought his gift of keys was only a logistical transaction to facilitate our renewed intimacy. But now I realized that it was far more: he was attempting to reverse his request for the return of his keys in 2013. The symbolism left me gobsmacked. I was moved. But I feared our opposite communication styles might run aground.

Gradually, we settled into a rhythm. Wednesday nights were our date nights; Friday and Saturday, Lars stayed over at my house.

We'd both been sleeping alone for years so sleeping through the night with a partner was a major adjustment. Given that I now had Lars's keys, I needed him to have my back. Literally. Our current mattresses transferred motion and didn't accommodate two light sleepers.

Within a few weeks, we were shopping for new beds.

Lars took charge, and by the end of January, we had a new California king bed with a Tempurpedic mattress and an adjustable frame with two remote control units that adjusted both head and foot which he had installed at his apartment. I got a new queen-size Tempurpedic. So, wherever we perched for the night, we were more comfortable.

We kept harkening back to 2013, reframing our history, marveling over how improbable it was that we'd reunited. By mid-February with unbounded optimism and a touch of madness, we decided to move in together.

We agreed to look for a four-bedroom place where we could fit the two new beds, plus room for two home offices. Besides sleep and sex, work was a priority.

Bay Area rents were over the moon. We looked at a place in the Oakland hills that had amazing views of the bay and the city but had only two closets in two thousand square feet and no garage. There was the lovely four-bedroom house in Berkeley where the two basement bedrooms were encrusted with mold and the kitchen had a ceramic rooster backsplash and cabinets circa 1954. Or the townhouse on Bay Farm Island, walkable to the ferry to San Francisco, but with an elementary school playground behind the backyard fence. Not one of these could be had for less than four thousand dollars a month.

We had crashed headlong into a wall of affordability. For two months we searched. Prices continued to escalate. In desperation, we decided to look on the other side of the Caldecott Tunnel, the "wormhole" as one friend called it because when you moved east to Contra Costa County, you entered a different reality.

I had been making payments on the pearl and diamond ring that I'd put on layaway at my favorite jewelers. I asked Lars if he'd go with me to pick it up. It was late April and my birthday in mid-May was barreling toward us. It was time.

Lars took my hand as we walked to the store, a short block from where we had parked. When we reached Janko's double glass doors there was a large sign that read, "Close Out Sale: 40 Percent Off."

Lars grinned.

"I didn't know they were closing," I said.

"It's our lucky day," he said.

I had told him about getting engaged to myself. Inside, as we waited for the owner to retrieve the little Manilla envelope with my ring inside, we browsed the glass cabinets. So much bling! It was dizzying.

She returned, pulled the ring out of the envelope, polished it, and set it on a velvet tray. It was even more gorgeous than I remembered.

Lars stared down at the dozens of rings displayed in the case. The owner asked if she could show him something else.

He turned to me.

"See anything you like?"

I held my breath. If you're standing in a jewelry store next to a man you love in front of a tray of diamond rings and he asks you a question like that, well, what was I supposed to do?

I pointed at a white gold band encircled with diamond chips. Margo pulled it out of the case. I slipped it on my ring finger.

She beckoned for my hand. She slipped the engagement ring over the wedding band. They matched perfectly. I looked at Lars.

"I love it," I said.

He nodded his approval. "Now, I need a ring too," he said.

I gave him a searching look, but he appeared unphased. I was beginning to expect that Lars would surprise me; even so, I hadn't seen this coming.

Margo scanned the case, then selected a white gold band with a diamond chip in the center. She handed me the ring, and I turned to Lars and put it on his finger.

"I guess it's time to make an honest man of you," I said.

Margo said she needed to size the rings and asked if we wanted them engraved.

"We'll think about that and get back to you," Lars said.

I walked out of Janko's with a pearl and diamond ring on my left hand, one I had chosen for myself five months earlier, one I'd half-paid for. Lars paid for the other half. Instead of getting engaged to myself, I was at least half-engaged to Lars, who, without any discussion, had just written a very large check for the three rings.

"What a deal," I said as we left the store. "We got those rings for half price!"

"Okay then, 2018!" Lars grinned. "Hey, that's what we should put on our bands," he added.

I nodded my agreement. "Genius!"

We walked away from Janko's holding hands, giggling like a couple of seventh graders who'd just agreed to go steady. What would happen next? If Lars had a plan, he wasn't letting me in on it.

CHAPTER 14
ENGAGED

An errand that consisted of paying off the balance and picking up my ring had morphed into something much more—sort of like the keys in the gift bag. But this was more than symbolism. We appeared to be engaged.

I texted my daughter Greta a picture of the ring on my left hand.

She sent back a googly-eyed emoji. "Mom, are you engaged?!!"

I think so, I texted back. *He bought the ring, but he hasn't proposed.*

More emojis and exclamation marks.

Lars drove us to a Kiwanis gathering that was held at the Balena Bay Yacht Club in Alameda. As we walked the gangplank onto the boat deck and faced a phalanx of his friends, he beamed. It was as if our chance encounter with a sale we could not resist was Manifest Destiny.

"This is my fiancé, Eleanor," he said to one unsuspecting pal. The woman gasped.

Then he took my hand and began showing off the ring. Someone grabbed a bottle of Prosecco, filled two plastic cups, and handed them to us. We toasted by clinking glasses and sloshing Prosecco on the polished wooden floors of a forty-six-foot sailboat.

"I'm so happy for you," one of Lars's oldest woman friends said, leaning in confidentially. "You two are good for each other."

The men back-slapped and teased Lars. The women wanted to know if we had set a date. I demurred, stammering about how it was all so new and unexpected.

Had Lars intended to ask me to marry him simply because he bought my ring?

Was he planning to propose?

It seemed best to go with the flow. So, I acted as if it was a done deal, accepted the congratulations, and got mildly drunk on Prosecco. I knew that Lars would do things at his own pace and in his own way. The smart move was to let him.

The next day, we decided to walk around Lake Merritt and enjoy dinner at the Lake Chalet, a relatively new addition to the Oakland restaurant scene.

It was a gorgeous April afternoon, Earth Day weekend. The sky spread like a blue tea cozy over the lake. Hipsters pranced along with designer dogs dressed in little sweaters, bikers, and walkers vied for the right of way on the paths, and the sound of conga drums echoed from the colonnade at the north end of the lake.

Lake Chalet had originally been the municipal boat house for the city of Oakland. It was a crumbling eyesore until a developer bought it and turned it into a restaurant with expansive windows, views to die for, and a "Taco Tuesday" happy hour on the dock.

It also had a small gift shop with expensive blown glass tchotchkes and a gondola rental. The gondolas were authentic

Venetian models with carved wooden prows and ornate brass seahorses on the oarlocks.

As we approached the restaurant, Lars squeezed my hand.

"How about a gondola ride?"

"That sounds like fun," I said with a nonchalance I didn't feel.

Had he picked this romantic activity to ask me to marry him? My heart began to gallop.

After the proprietor swiped Lars's card through the machine, we waited on the dock for a gondola. I turned the unfamiliar ring back and forth on my finger using the thumb of my left hand. It felt like wiggling a loose tooth.

Once onboard, the gondolier handed us a parasol, which we took turns holding to shade ourselves from the late afternoon sun. Because of Earth Day and the fine weather, the dock was packed with people.

The gondolier promised that he would serenade us with authentic Italian songs. He poled out into open water, then used the huge oar to circumnavigate the south end of the lake. From there, you could see the Oakland hills, the colonnade, the Cathedral of Christ the Light, and even the building where I had worked until 2015. It was glorious!

Meanwhile, he belted out "Volare," and then "Arrivederci Roma" followed by a rousing chorus of "O Solo Mio" with operatic force.

Each time Lars took my hand, the gondolier began a new aria.

For half an hour, we exchanged meaningful glances, but words were impossible.

As our irrepressible songster oared us back toward the restaurant, someone on the dock shouted to us, "You guys look so happy!"

People broke into applause, assuming there had been a proposal. Lars looked jolly in his straw fedora. I wore a pearl pendant he had gotten me as a gift, a precursor to the rings. We sheltered under our pink parasol as we took in the shouts, but I was happy to disembark.

During dinner, I had a gnawing feeling that Lars might never propose. I worried that I'd never have the satisfaction of being asked for my hand.

Lying in bed next to him that night, I couldn't bear it any longer. Did he want to marry me or not?

To use a technical term, I had an "insecure attachment" to my mother; and my father was abusive. I was a needy, insecure child who masked her feelings of rejection with pretend confidence, a trait I carried into adulthood. I was desperate for concrete evidence that Lars wanted me.

"I need you to say the words," I whispered.

By now it had been twenty-four hours since we'd purchased the rings. We'd been serenaded in a gondola. People on the dock had clapped for us. I was wearing my new ring with its lustrous pearl and sparkly diamonds and sharing pictures on Facebook. But I still had not received a proposal of marriage. All the hoopla might be a road to nowhere.

"You mean, get down on one knee and all that?" Lars didn't whisper. His voice boomed through the dark room.

"Yes," I said. "And all that."

"Do you want me to propose in a baseball stadium, or get down on one knee in a restaurant?"

"No! I have a horror of public proposals. But I need you to ask me."

The next morning, I went to the kitchen to brew tea. Suddenly, I sensed Lars behind me. I turned. He stood there naked except for his plaid boxers. Then, he dropped to one knee on the tile floor, put both hands on my waist, and said, "Eleanor, will you marry me?"

My first impulse was to help him up. We were too old for this!

But it was so touching, so chivalrous, and so perfectly Lars.

I put one hand on his shoulder, as if I were about to knight him. With as much solemnity as I could muster, I said, "Yes, Lars. I will marry you."

He lifted himself from his knees. We hugged. The teakettle whistled. We were officially engaged. It didn't happen in any of the expected places—the jewelry store, the yacht, the gondola with the caterwauling gondolier, or the restaurant. Lars sculpted the moment himself without relying on fairytales, or 1940s movie scenes.

It was an original get-down-on-your-knees moment, bowed before your lady love, dressed only in your underwear to ask for her hand in marriage.

Hell yes, I thought to myself. *And about time too.*

CHAPTER 15
WHAT I LEFT OUT

1. Greta and Jim bought a four-bedroom house and moved to West Sacramento in July of 2017, with seven-year-old Zoe and Amelia, about to turn four. I was happy for their good fortune but brokenhearted. Up until then, I was an active, involved grandmother. I missed them all terribly. By August I was looking for a house in Sacramento. I imagined becoming a gypsy, finding a cottage where I could flit away from Oakland and start over. By October, I had come to my senses. Still brokenhearted, I decided that my friends, my work, and the life I had carefully crafted were worth preserving. For me, writing was like breathing and I needed all the oxygen I could get. And I suspected that moving closer would make Greta feel crowded, so I quietly shelved my plans.

2. When Greta left town with her family, the sense of loss flooded me with memories of my older daughter Maya's sudden death. But I could not fully admit the depth of my grief. I was so invested in being "better" after losing my firstborn, in having survived her loss. I was proud of how I'd been able to go on for twenty-five years without her.

Proud of all the spiritual and psychological work I had done. Crumbling in the face of my surviving daughter being a functional, talented, successful adult—in the face of her leaving me—was a defeat I could not tolerate. That was the depression trigger, the beginning of the quicksand I fell into in the fall of 2017. So, when Lars reappeared, I was looking for a hand out of that pit, and he extended his.

3. I had long known that I'd take Lars back if he'd let me. His steadiness was calming, almost soporific. I needed it the same way the neighborhood cats needed the catnip I grew in a pot by my front door. A parade of felines pranced onto my patio, rubbed against the catnip leaves, rolled on their backs, paws pointing skyward, and celebrated their cat lives, high as coke fiends, rubbing and rolling, making low happy growling noises. Lars's deep stillness had a similar effect on me.

4. In 2009, I dated a brilliant physicist who was bipolar and didn't reliably take his meds. He once asked me what I was addicted to, what I couldn't live without. He said that for him gambling was a high he could not resist. Then he squinted at me through wire-rimmed glasses, and said, "You are a love addict." The moment those words rolled out, I vibrated with their truth. A bolt of shame split open some locked place in my chest. A few weeks later we got into an awful fight. He slammed his fist on my coffee table and leaned toward me as if he might strike me. It scared me sober. I went straight to a Sex and Love Addicts Anonymous meeting. I went weekly. I found a temporary sponsor; the meeting was so oversubscribed there were no permanent sponsors. I practiced sober

dating and didn't have sex for the next three years and ten months.

5. Lars was the first man I thought I could maintain emotional sobriety with after my long period of celibacy. I delayed having sex with him for three months, a long time for an addict. He was patient, and emotionally neutral, which mystified me, but also felt safe. With Lars, there was a chance I could maintain enough sobriety to choose consciously, and not be swept away, not fall into old patterns. He was my opposite, someone who operated in such a blank emotional field that he almost floated. In therapy speak, this is called hypoarousal. I was typically on the ragged edge of hyperarousal, primed to escalate my emotions in roller coaster waves at a moment's notice. When things went well, we met in the middle. With Lars, I began to understand that an even keel was possible.

6. In December of 2017, I became a temporary foster mom for a Maine Coon cat. I intended to keep him for the holidays, and then return him. Marlowe was from Cat Town. They rescued cats that were too old, too feral, or too ill and would be killed by the city shelter. Lucky for me, he was healthy, although he was considered a senior cat at the age of eight, and he was highly anxious from having bounced from one temporary home to another. He had gnawed off a huge chunk of fur on one of his flanks and had a bald patch, but he was otherwise the most handsome cat I'd ever seen. He had a white ruff and white paws the size of mini muffins. When I let him out of his carrier, I expected him to run under the bed and hide. Instead, he began exploring my living room while "trilling," a questioning meow peculiar to Maine Coons, as if he wanted

to understand where he was and who I was, and what would happen next. We started a conversation. I'd say something. He'd reply. Then he'd trill another question at me. Within five minutes, I said right out loud, "Dude! You are not going anywhere." I was in love.

7. Days later, my encounter with Lars mirrored how I felt about finding Marlowe. And as with Marlowe, I didn't want to let him go.

8. Lars would hold Marlowe under his front legs and dance him back and forth so that Marlowe's giant paws waggled from side to side. He rubbed Marlowe's head with abandon, in a way most cats would never tolerate. Marlowe would go and sit on Lars's belly when he was napping on the couch, rising and falling with my beloved's breath, like a Disneyland ride. As time passed, they grew ever closer. I could never trust a man who didn't love my cat.

9. It happened when my mother was bent over the kitchen sink, washing dishes, her body arched as if bowing to the dirty dishes. As if she was begging the dishes to forgive her, to love her, her unshed tears piling up in the rinse water. I was fifteen, and only a few weeks before I had discovered Mom was a lesbian by walking in on her and her lover. I love-hated my mother. She would sometimes lash out at me without warning or ignore my repeated calls of "Mom" for hours. She never shielded me from my father. She had enlisted me to protect her secrets against my will. My feet felt rooted to the linoleum, although I wanted out of there in the worst way. Perched precariously in the dish drainer was a carving knife, its blade worn thin from decades of carving Sunday roasts. I could see myself leaping across the kitchen. Grabbing the knife.

Plunging the blade into my mother's back, a parenthesis of blood seeping through her white cotton shirt. But I pulled down the blinds in my head. I shut the door and slammed it on my crazy thoughts.

10. As a teenager, I'd concluded that my mother subconsciously pushed me in front of my father so that I could take the abuse instead of her. I hated her for not protecting me. I resented the way she leaned into her victim status and used it to make me feel sorry for her as if being a doormat made her saintly. The pattern continued. Once, after an abusive boyfriend had given me a black eye, she urged me to date him again when he came to the house to beg me to go out. She said it right in front of him: "Ellie, you can't just shut him out, you have to give him another chance." She had a knack for enabling violence while ducking any blame for it. When I did go out with him because my mother undermined my attempt to say no, he tried to strangle me because I refused to have sex with him.

11. In real life, I've participated in euthanizing several animals, and each time I think I won't be able to do it because I love them too much. When the suffering of an animal is unbearable, it becomes imperative to release them. We say it's the "humane" thing to do. Yet when doctors give a dying patient too much morphine, we judge them harshly. I wanted to relieve myself of my mother's misery and stop the drama of her unceasing victimhood. Would that have been a mercy killing? Or just an extreme way to separate myself from her? Finding my way apart from my mother was a Sisyphean task that lasted decades, one I'm still not sure I've completed.

12. In my twenties, I moved 2,500 hundred miles away, as far as I could go from my fractured family, and still be on the same continent. Greta moved fifty-six miles away to West Sacramento. I guess I should count myself lucky. By the time she was eighteen, I knew that she knew how to get separate, that she was making a clean break. But I sometimes still wondered about her anger, her unspoken grievances. They manifest in little verbal jabs, in long silences between visits. Could I be imagining that? I'm afraid to ask her.

13. My granddaughters Zoe and Amelia have cats named Mochi and Ozzie. These two cats fight, sometimes brutally. Ozzie is male; he must be the alpha. He's black and sleek and playful. Mochi is more sensitive, and of course, she's the girl cat. He attacks her, jumps on her back, and hisses at her. Sometimes she'll defend herself. Sometimes she disappears. After Ozzie mauled a hummingbird, Amelia held a funeral for the bird, and in the middle of the ceremony, the bird sat up and flew away.

CHAPTER 16
MALE BIRD, FEMALE BIRD

When 2018 began, I was single, living on Erie Street in my Oakland condo looking out at the hills above Lakeshore Avenue. Lars had a two-bedroom bachelor pad, a place I fondly called "The Dust Palace."

Three weeks after our engagement, I turned seventy. Three days after that, a moving van stood outside my door. Life barreled forward at a velocity I dimly remembered from my twenties.

During this move from single to coupled, from my own space to a rented condo in a Walnut Creek retirement community, my mind overflowed with details and logistics: Missing curtain rods, a bathtub drain that wouldn't close, Marlowe's sharp nails desperately in need of a trim, a garage full of boxes, forwarded mail. Dismantling my old life was like an echo in a funhouse tunnel. It kept on going and going, driving me mad!

In 1978, a psychic had told me that moving cross-country from Worthington, Minnesota to Nevada City, California was akin to taking a file drawer full of folders and dumping them out on the floor. Scraps of my old life flung about in a messy heap. At that time, I was joining my life with a man as well, the man who became my second husband.

As I unpacked boxes, I flashed back to that spring when we left Minnesota and drove west to California. We crossed the Sierra Nevada mountains in a blizzard, the Oldsmobile creeping toward Donner Summit, the scrape of the windshield wipers hauling slush from side to side, my five-year-old asleep in the backseat with her favorite blanket and her doll. It was April Fool's Day. The snow lashed me, mocking my decision to sell our snow shovels because I thought we were going to a warm sunny place.

When we finally reached the rented cabin on Banner Mountain and all I wanted was a hot bath, I discovered two large frogs in the bathtub, inside a freezing bathroom that had been added to the cabin as a sloppy afterthought.

I was about to turn thirty and there was so much life still to live; now, I was taking another gamble, a merger with a man who was my total opposite. I comforted myself with the thought that it wasn't snowing, at least, and that no one else would have to bear the results of my decision, certainly not my little daughter.

I hoped I'd learned a thing or two since then.

Lars and I went through the wormhole of the Caldecott Tunnel and rented a condo in Rossmoor at the end of a leafy cul de sac. Surprisingly, Rossmoor was more affordable than anything we had looked at in Oakland or Berkeley. Still, we were skeptical. Did we want to live in a gated community restricted to residents over the age of fifty-five? But we liked the layout of the condo, it had room for two home offices, and the rent was reasonable.

The movers carried in box after box, stacking them in every room. Then came the sofa, the media stand, the desks, and the furniture for the guest bedroom. At a moment of maximum chaos, Marlowe saw his chance. He gave us the slip and raced into the sideyard. At that exact moment, a deer streaked down the hill toward the house. Never having seen such a large fast-moving animal before, Marlowe bolted. The deer freaked out. They disappeared into the shrubs on the hillside behind the condo, two blurs slamming toward the horizon.

"You should have kept him in the carrier," the woman I'd hired to help me organize the kitchen said. "Cats hate having their territory disrupted."

I nodded, humbly pretending I should have known better, when in fact, I did know better. I thought Marlowe was safely secured in the guest bedroom.

I asked Lars to go out and hunt for him. I kept unwrapping plates and glasses, neatly folding packing paper, and using an X-Acto knife to slit cardboard boxes and flatten them.

Later, after the kitchen was put together, I went out to search. I called and called, walking up and down our entry, the long common driveway that led from one four-unit building to the next. Huge oak trees spun circular shadows as a late afternoon breeze stirred their canopies. Above our entry was a hillside with fields of wild mustard whipping back and forth in the wind.

"Damn! I'm in the country!"

Free from unpacking, I found myself surrounded by glorious nature.

A flock of wild turkeys wove through the wild mustard and crossed the road above the entry. They strutted, officious as small-town mayors, looking as if they owned the place.

I came home empty-handed. Marlowe was still at large. Lars ordered takeout for dinner, and we ate pasta and salad on our newly unpacked plates at our newly set up dining room table. We fell into bed at ten o'clock exhausted.

"Honey, are you awake?" It was two o'clock in the morning and I thought I'd heard a plaintiff meow.

"I am now," Lars responded, more groggy than grumpy.

He threw on his jeans and stumbled out to look. Five minutes later he was back with Marlowe under his arm. He had been sitting on our neighbor's porch, calling for us.

With help from two professionals and several friends, the house was put together and functioning. Most of my things were hung or shelved in logical places. Our glorious king-size bed lorded over our new bedroom.

Lars took a different approach. He moved four boxes at a time, crammed with dust-covered household items, not taped shut or labeled, in the back of his station wagon. He had not given notice or vacated his old apartment. Each day he went to retrieve more.

He painstakingly disassembled bookshelves—seven of them, each six feet tall—hauling them out of the car and stacking the orphaned shelves in our new living room with the screws taped to the shelves. Then he'd drive back through the Caldecott Tunnel for more belongings.

To make room for the bookshelves, he emptied the contents of his home office from our den. Computer monitors, keyboards, and random cords burst from plastic shopping bags; stacks of folders and papers stuck out at odd angles from boxes that overflowed into the living room I had so carefully arranged. For an entire weekend, I walked by, breath held, eyes averted, heart pounding until he moved everything back inside the den and closed his office door.

"To the most *dis*unorganized person I know ..." my seventh-grade Civics teacher, Mr. Healey, had written to me. Finally, I fully understood his blue ballpoint scrawl in the margin of my yearbook.

Disorder breeds panic in my inner child. She thinks she's back in a Pennsylvania farmhouse in a maelstrom of emotional chaos. Mr. Healey saw that my organization was a reaction, my neatness a coping mechanism. Order and beauty helped that little girl feel safer.

Lars was precisely the opposite. Books piled on every surface, computer cables dangling from boxes, and stacks of paper spilling across his desk spelled home to him.

"The very thing that keeps me sane makes you crazy and vice versa," I said.

He just nodded and went back to hanging pictures, carefully measuring each space, putting blue masking tape where the nails should go, and making sure our "his and hers" art collection was displayed harmoniously on our walls.

Over many weeks, and after many fights, we built a shared space. With each book and fork, each dish towel and pot holder—with every decision—we painstakingly created a new life.

Once we settled, it was only a matter of time before our opposite needs—his for clutter, mine for order—clashed. There may be couples in which the messy one is the woman, but I honestly cannot picture it.

There's a Nicole Hollander cartoon in which Harry the bartender asks Sylvia how she can tell a caged male bird from his mate, the female bird.

Sylvia responds: "He's the one with the furrowed brow; she's the happy-go-lucky one."

Harry: "Be serious."

Sylvia: "He's the one reading the sports page; she's the one with twelve pairs of tiny shoes."

I lined up my twelve pairs of tiny shoes neatly on pull-out racks in my closet. Lars scattered his shoes under the bench by our front door. I cut a deal with him. His office and the garage loft were his territory—he could fill them with dusty computer equipment and back tax forms, and I would not complain.

Our truce lasted for a few weeks until, imperceptibly, the lower garage began to fill with random canvas bags of junk, as if carried in by malevolent elves. When I couldn't stand it any longer, I put my foot down. But over time, I learned, the clutter inevitably reappeared.

In the end, three months after we moved in, Lars vacated his old apartment. He stored the rest of his hoard in two storage units, a few miles from his old place. He refused to get rid of anything. Even our financial planner tried to convince him he didn't have the luxury of paying to store stuff he'd never use. But Lars was unmoved. He clung to old cardboard boxes stuffed with broken computer parts, shirts worthy of the Goodwill, CDs and DVDs from prior decades; dusty remnants of his old life.

CHAPTER 17
REALLY?

We negotiated our shared space, attempting to adjust to each other and our wildly different environment. No need for a date night on Wednesdays now that we were living together. As June rolled around, lovemaking dwindled from a guaranteed weekend activity to a tentative every-other-week event.

We went on a two-week vacation and never had sex. I was upset and mystified, but I rationalized it with a jest.

"We are the only couple on the face of the planet who never made love on vacation."

"Really?"

He looked at me with furled eyebrows, as if this hadn't occurred to him.

Several weeks later, I'd had enough. As we lingered over dinner, and finally pushed our plates away, I said, "What is wrong with us?"

He stared straight ahead, his face blank.

"I mean..." I began again. "Why don't we have sex anymore?"

By now, the boxes had been unpacked, the hundreds of books shelved, the art hung—a major undertaking since we combined our paintings—and somehow, we'd gotten through all that. But week by week, we were becoming more like friendly room-mates, and less like formerly passionate lovers. Was it our ages? Proximity? Declining libido?

That night, as we talked, it dawned on me that this was our new normal. That fast red car we'd climbed into in January had hurtled to the bottom of the hill and crashed into an embank-ment. We were out of gas, stalled in our new-old relationship, navigating without a map.

Day by day intimacy drained out of our relationship. If Lars was concerned, he didn't show it. I kept trying. I wanted to get to the bottom of whatever was driving us apart. Each time I tried to discuss it, he shut me down. At times our talks ended in me bursting into tears and Lars storming off to his office. We were at an impasse.

I began obsessively researching autism spectrum disorder, especially from the neurotypical partner's point of view. Back at the beginning of dating Lars, I had suspected Asperger's. Now, I started to take it seriously. I read books by Maxine Aston and Rudy Simone, and articles by experts like Tony Atwood and Simon Baron-Cohen. I combed the internet for information on neurodivergence in relationships. I was desperate to find out why our love life had dropped off a cliff, and Lars couldn't tell me.

"Is Lars okay?" Greta looked concerned.

We had driven to West Sacramento that morning. Lars went to troubleshoot some computer issues at a branch office of the Bay Area company where he worked. I spent the afternoon with my granddaughters.

When he returned, we were in Greta's kitchen making snacks for the girls. The front door opened and shut, but Lars never appeared.

I found him asleep in the guest bedroom, snoring softly.

By now, I had learned to anticipate abrupt disappearances. Many evenings, he would vanish without saying goodnight. He'd be sound asleep when I came to bed.

"This is normal behavior for him," I told my daughter. "If he gets tired or overwhelmed, he disappears and goes to sleep."

When she had first met Lars in 2013, Greta told me that she felt there was something not quite right, that he didn't make eye contact, and couldn't stay on topic in our dinner conversation, and that he seemed more interested in impressing her than in connecting.

Now, I blurted out "I think he's on the autism spectrum."

She shot me a look. Greta was the first person I'd talked to about my observations, other than my therapist and Lars himself.

"Has he been diagnosed?"

"No. I don't think he wants to be," I said.

An hour later, Lars emerged, jolly and sociable. I decided to go with the flow. Later, as we prepared for bed, I reminded him that as a guest it was considered bad form to simply disappear. Perhaps he could have come in, said hello, and excused himself for a rest.

"I hear what you're saying," he said.

Then he turned over, pulled up the covers, and went to sleep. I lay awake wondering what to do. He may have heard me, but did he understand? I felt caught in the middle, trying to explain Lars to others when I didn't understand him myself.

I got up and left Lars asleep in the guest room. I put on my robe and went into the kitchen. We had brought Marlowe with us. He rubbed my ankles as I put out food for him.

Zoe was on the couch playing a game on her iPad. Greta and Jim were asleep. Amelia was in the kid's playroom watching a movie.

"Hi, Zoe. Do you want some toast?"

She glanced up and nodded. I busied myself by finding bread, butter, and jam.

Lars came in, dressed in his customary black jeans and long-sleeve shirt. He declined my offer of toast but said yes to a cup of tea.

I brought the tea and toast to the table. Zoe sat side by side with Lars on the couch. Lars had a large store of riddles in his brain, and he posed one to her.

Marlowe sat between them. Zoe began to pet him as she considered the riddle and then played with his large white paws. She lifted him to her chest for a hug. He squirmed away.

"Don't do that!" Lars said.

"Why not?"

"Because he doesn't like it."

"Yes, he does."

Marlowe had fled and was lying under the coffee table.

Zoe chanted like a broken record, "He does too like it! He does too!" Then she poked Lars in the side.

He grabbed her arm. She struggled, at first giggling. Then she told him to stop.

"You're hurting me," she said.

"Hey, you two! Knock it off!" I was standing at the table.

My fiancé and my nine-year-old granddaughter went at each other like playground rivals. Before I could step in, Lars leaned over. Still gripping Zoe's arm, he put his mouth to her wrist.

I was stunned. I half doubted my own eyes.

Zoe began to cry. She rubbed her wrist. "He bit me," she wailed.

I went to her. She extended her hand. A circle of faint red marks stood out on the skin but hadn't broken it.

I turned on Lars. "What were you thinking?"

"I was trying to show her what would happen if she kept bothering Marlowe."

"By *biting* her?"

"She has to learn..." he trailed off.

Hugging Zoe to my side, I stood up, led her to the dining room table, pulled out her chair, and sat her down in front of her toast.

I turned to Lars. "You need a time-out," I said. "That is not okay."

He hunched into himself on the sofa, not meeting my eyes.

I sat down at the table, heart pounding. I spread jam on Zoe's toast.

Lars left the living room as silently as a ghost through the sliding door to the patio. I could see him from the dining room windows, calmly reading a magazine at the patio table, as if nothing out of the ordinary had happened.

I turned to Zoe. "Are you okay?"

She had a pile of crusts on her plate. She pushed one to the side, then nodded.

"I'm sorry," I said. "I'm sure he didn't mean it."

Greta and Jim had planned a romantic getaway to celebrate their wedding anniversary. I had agreed that Lars and I would stay with the kids while they went away overnight. I'd explained to my daughter about the bite mark on Zoe's wrist and apologized on my beloved's behalf. Zoe seemed to have forgotten the incident already, and if Greta had doubts about our watching the kids, she didn't express them.

Lars went off to work at the branch office again. Peace returned. After Jim came home from work, the three of us sat outside at their patio table watching Zoe and Amelia practice underwater flips in the pool. We were all in our bathing suits.

I had brought presents for their anniversary and the table was scattered with gift bags and tissue. A bottle of Prosecco was sweating in an ice bucket nearby. We were going out to dinner at a nearby restaurant, so Greta called the kids to get out of the pool.

We were deep in conversation when the slider opened, and Lars came out.

"Hi Lars, want a beer?" Jim and Lars shared a passion for craft brews.

"How did your work go?" I asked.

"Okay," he said. "I solved a couple of problems."

Jim brought the beer. The sun lasered through the orange umbrella above the table, and the cement patio shimmered with reflected heat. Greta and I turned back to our conversation.

When I looked up again, Lars had taken a purple gift bag from the table and pulled it down over his head. He sat with a glass of IPA in front of him looking like SpongeBob Square Pants minus the googly eyes, a large flat purple square where his face should have been.

It reminded me of when I would cover my face with my hands as a three-year-old and declare, "You can't see me," as if I were invisible. But Lars sat there, his head inside a purple bag, visible as fuck.

I shrank back in the chair cushions, trying to disappear myself, pretending this wasn't happening. Heat gathered into a ball in my brain, paralysis spreading through me.

The three of us exchanged puzzled looks. What could I possibly say?

After a few minutes, Lars took the bag off his head, folded it neatly, and began drinking his beer. No one said a word about it; I reasoned it was better not to give this odd behavior any more attention. I tried to imagine what motivated him, but I was mystified.

The girls lollygagged for as long as they could, but at last, got out of the pool and dried off. The grownups went to freshen up. The kids put on sundresses and brushed their hair.

Dinner at a nearby restaurant was torture. Lars was surly and unresponsive despite valiant attempts to bring him into the conversation. I was mortally embarrassed.

I asked myself, "Do I have the strength for this?"

The next day as I fixed food for the kids, cleaned up the kitchen, and helped them get dressed, Lars vanished into his laptop, then into a book. We barely spoke the entire day. I was furious and lonely. I had no idea how to talk about what had happened, or even how to talk at all.

I kept asking myself, *Really? Did that really happen?*

"I can forgive a lot," I told my therapist in our next session. "But I don't think I can ever forgive Lars for biting my granddaughter. Who does that?"

"Someone with a lot of undigested trauma," she replied.

CHAPTER 18
HOW WE GOT HERE

Lars sat across from me at the dinner table, silent as a stone. I had finally made a direct request: please go to couples counseling with me.

"If we don't get some help, we're not going to make it as a couple. And that would be too sad." Tears pricked the back of my eyes.

"We love each other. We have the ways, the means, the resources. I'm not giving up."

After an on-again, off-again conversation stretching over several days, Lars agreed. I called the counseling center at Rossmoor and made an appointment.

※

In the end, are all intimate relationships a power struggle? That's what books say. I think maybe it's deeper, more complicated, as when you stand by a frozen lake and see the dark patches of water beneath, the places where the ice could crack. Do you trust and drive your car out to the middle, chop a hole in the ice, and drop in a line? Or, like me, do you stand back and watch, wait for the slow rumble of the fracture, and be glad you're still standing on the bank?

I'm always testing. Looking for love to be proven. Maybe that lack of trust is about power or the illusion of control. It's also about wanting the bond to be real and strong.

In my college psychology textbook, there was a picture of a baby monkey clinging to a terrycloth mother monkey, its little paws wrapped around the wire frame in a death grip. As a 19-year-old, I stared at that picture for a long time. I recognized that longing in myself. The need to attach. To be comforted. To cling, if necessary.

I wanted to reach into that photo and pluck that little monkey out and cuddle it against my heart. I wanted to be that monkey being cuddled. I wanted someone to hold me to his heart. It was too late for me and my mother. She too had stood by the bank, watching, not dropping in her line, not committing. She was so scarred, so scared. She couldn't touch us, her children. At the end of her life, my mother would not let me hug her for longer than twenty seconds. She had been sexually abused by a teacher when she was a preteen and never recovered. To her, intimate touch was an electric shock, a cattle prod.

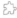

When I decided to move in with Lars, I figured I knew what I was getting into. In the "before time," I knew that he was a hoarder. His bachelor pad was a mess. He had books stacked to the ceiling, the bookshelves overflowed, and his collection of CDs and DVDs sat in teetering piles or three deep on shelves. There was a huge potted plant, fronds stretched out like arms, sitting in the middle of the kitchen stove because he never cooked.

When I peered into his fridge there would be a jar of olives, some sort of designer ale or lager, and a hunk of cheese with its edges ripening to green.

But for some reason, I thought we had made an agreement. We had talked it over.

"The things that comfort you give me an anxiety attack," I had said when this so-called agreement was being negotiated. "I have to have order in my space."

He had nodded and given me his Yoda "what will be, will be" grin. I took that for agreement. He'd get an office where he could do whatever he wanted with his stuff if he kept the door closed, and I'd generously give him the extra storage in the garage's attic where he could pile up old electronics and power cords to his heart's content. But the house would be organized to my standards.

One evening, I was meticulously editing the closets and organizing my dresser drawers. I heard a clunk, clunk, clunk, like the sound of a refrigerator being delivered. I went to check. The door scraped open.

Lars stood in the entry balancing a black metal dolly piled high with open boxes of dust-laden books. Books that went back to the Pleistocene—his time at a liberal arts college where he did nothing but read and discuss the great books. He read about the Peloponnesian Wars, and all of Homer, works in Latin and ancient Greek, plus all of Shakespeare's plays. I gulped.

"Hi honey," I said, holding back a "WTF" comment, practically choking on it. Was our agreement about how we would co-exist in our new space a figment of my imagination?

"Hi," Lars said. He began unloading boxes from the dolly and stacking them helter-skelter in the living room. Dust motes hung in the air as if we were standing in Heracleum, transported to ancient times, and volcanic ash was raining down. It smelled like death.

"Lars, I thought we agreed you would keep any books that didn't fit in your new office in storage." I had the tiniest smidgeon of doubt. That is what we said, isn't it?

"These will fit," he said.

I surveyed the growing piles of boxes. There were more books in plastic bags, overflowing. Our beautifully organized living room was reverting to chaos.

The ongoing muddle of our day-to-day life was a Tiramisu cake with layers of different colored emotions, shames, withdrawals, evasions, and self-justifications.

Lars is afraid, I realized when he said at one of our therapy sessions that if he felt observed, he felt judged.

"He doesn't want to be seen!" It went off like an explosion in my brain.

Our therapist said, "That's very interesting," and then paused. "I hear you saying you don't like the feeling of being seen. But that's the essence of intimacy, being seen by your partner."

"Yes," I chimed in. "That's why relationships are so scary."

The silence that followed was like dropping a rock down a well, it took forever to hit bottom. Lars gazed at the far horizon and spoke not one word.

I realized during that interminable silence that I had the same fear. When Lars came into the kitchen while I was cooking and stood three feet away watching, I felt as if I might jump out of my skin. That sense of being watched and evaluated carried me back in time to the moment when my father appraised my ten-year-old body as I was on my way out the door to play and said, completely out of the blue, "Your rear end sticks out like a bustle."

A child's bottom is a private place, especially for a girl on the cusp of womanhood. I wanted to drop under our house and hide. I froze with my hand on the doorknob. Part of me was still frozen, waiting for the next cutting comment, the punch I didn't see coming, the critique.

I looked at the therapist and reminded myself to breathe. I wasn't a child, trapped in an old house on Gusty Hill in a little Pennsylvania college town. I was here. It was now. And yet I knew, deep in my body, that I was every bit as afraid as Lars.

I wish I could say my realization made me philosophical, or capable of more understanding. Or that I could figure out the meaning inside my silent partner's thoughts. What I took away from that therapy session was the centrality of fear. How it shaped us like waves hitting rock, the rock of our little child souls moving through time. We both felt it. Those two little children on their separate islands, afraid and alone, not knowing how to find each other.

Much as I wanted to connect with Lars, much as I loved him, I felt frozen with fear. I wanted to say, "I see you and it's okay to be afraid. I feel the same."

But somehow the words never came.

More than any other year of my life, 2018 barreled ahead like a speeding train driven by the sorcerer's apprentice. There were moments when self-doubt—or realistic caution—warned my logical left brain that I was moving awfully fast, that Lars operated on a different wavelength.

Throughout three decades of being single with occasional longer-term relationships, I had longed for more permanence and a dependable companion. Once I'd given up hope, the dream materialized when Lars returned. And I did not want to give up on my dream. My heart and my right brain won the day.

I doubled down. After escrow closed on my old place in Oakland, I immediately began to look for a new place. Northern California real estate is vexing beyond belief. But it had given me a measure of stability and accumulated wealth I never imagined I'd have as a single woman. Now that I had a partner, I wanted the same for him. I wanted a home for us.

Rentals at Rossmoor are time-limited. We had signed a one-year lease to test the water. The community was a little Shangri-La where people still greeted each other when they passed, read the weekly community newspaper, borrowed books from the Rossmoor library, and attended the free movies shown every week—a happy little time warp. We both loved living there, so I thought.

Although Lars had never owned a home, he had lived for nine years in a house owned by his second wife. When they split, he did not retain so much as custody of the dogs. She kept the house and he felt as if he had been put out on the curb with the week's garbage. I didn't want to repeat that trauma or have him feel as if he was renting from me.

Lars was making very good money managing databases and providing computer support for the small company where he worked. I had methodically climbed the real estate ladder in the Bay Area. We were well qualified to buy. We immediately began to search for a permanent home. After looking at more than three dozen Rossmoor condos, we found one we both loved.

Late in 2018, we closed escrow on the same model condo we'd been renting—two bedrooms with a den and enclosed patio, providing enough space for two home offices.

Lars was in the orbital pull of his iPad; the magnetic glow of the screen lit his face. From time to time, he bent over his toast, slathered with butter and marmalade, looking away from the screen for a moment to take a bite, then quickly diving back into the virtual realm.

Is this an autism thing, I wondered, *or just a guy thing?* I wondered that a lot. Lars read obsessively but rarely seemed to finish a book. I'd find little brass bookmarkers two-thirds of the way through the books he loaned me. Books rotated on his bedside table. He dipped into them for information, then extracted his concentration and lasered it elsewhere—usually on a scientific YouTube video or a nerdy TED talk.

"You're on the spectrum. You know that don't you?" I finally asked.

He only smiled.

When we reunited, I was bone-shatteringly lonely and so grateful to have Lars in my life again. I reasoned that we had built a friendship. I knew him. I suspected he was neurodivergent, but I told myself I could handle it. If he had diabetes or a heart condition, I reasoned, I'd find a way to support him. Why should an autism spectrum disorder be any different?

He was smart, dependable, and devoted to good works through Kiwanis, and he had wooed me with an ardor that won my heart. I was in love. He had a high-paying job that he loved. We had many interests in common. We were working things out in therapy. And now, at the dawn of 2019, we were homeowners. I plunged ahead with renewed optimism.

CHAPTER 19
WHAT ELSE I LEFT OUT

1. Like a mother bear, I stood on my hind legs and fought for love, fought to hold on to my dream, fought for that romantic vision of Ed and Nids kissing in their kitchen, fought to understand Lars's family and my family, two sets of opposite but equal dysfunction. In the imagined version of my life, I saw myself in a happy marriage with a partner who was loving and communicative. But in real life, my relationships with men always foundered on the rocks of partial communication, escalating to fights, and my jumping ship before the man in question could end it. I was determined that would not be my pattern with Lars. I made up my mind not to be defeated by our different brain wiring.

2. Our condo was painted gray-green, the color of plants after rain. We had an expansive view of the Las Trampas hills, surrounded by California oaks and tall evergreen trees. Before we moved in, we hired an electrician and upgraded the power to the current building code. We put ceiling fans and recessed eco-efficient lighting in the rooms and dimmer switches on all the fixtures. We

repainted the kitchen cabinets, created open shelving, installed under cabinet lighting, put new ceramic tile in the kitchen and entry hall, and repainted the entire house in a Benjamin Moore color called "sea mist," which sometimes reads pale gray, sometimes pale green. We made the perfect nest. Give Lars and me a list of tasks and no one does a better job of checking them off. Were we house proud? Damn straight! I didn't vacuum every day, though.

3. Rossmoor has more than two hundred and fifty social clubs. There's everything you can imagine from golf to ceramics to bocce ball, to political and investment clubs. You could be busy seven nights a week. I joined the Mindful Living Club and began daily meditation with a group of like-minded elders. I also became a member of Sustainable Rossmoor and lobbied for solar panels and electric vehicles. I joined Rossmoor Advocates for Diversity and stood on one of our main roads with hundreds of my fellow residents waving a sign that read "Do Better, America!" after George Floyd was murdered. I've attended more marches and rallies since 2016 than I did when I was in college at Baldwin-Wallace, only miles from the campus at Kent State where state troopers shot four anti-war student protesters.

4. Once we moved to Rossmoor, commuting to San Francisco to work at the Writers Grotto became a time-consuming slog. So, I joined a smaller co-working community in Berkeley called Left Margin Lit where I could find street parking and get home in half an hour. I still belong to the Grotto. Now, I go to twice the parties.

5. A Grotto colleague who had lived in Italy and spoke Italian fluently sent out a notice that she was renting a villa outside Lucca, Italy for a week and invited others to join. The deal included a private chef who would cook delicious meals and offer cooking lessons. She sent photos of the villa. It was owned by a Contessa, had an expansive yard and garden, high ceilings, and curving stairs, and was within walking distance of a Tuscan winery. It took me about five minutes to decide to sign up. Lars readily agreed. Since we'd be going to Tuscany, we'd have to visit Florence, and possibly include the Cinque Terre hill towns. As I planned the trip, I had a realization. "This is a honeymoon," I said to Lars. "Do you think we should get married?"

6. By May, we'd been engaged for a year. We'd gotten counseling. We'd settled into our new house. We'd filed our taxes. Our financial planner said we should go to the local courthouse and get married immediately. He knew of cases where Social Security benefits that should have gone to the surviving spouse could not be claimed after an unexpected death, and because Lars was younger than me, he could claim spousal benefits until he was ready to file for his own. We'd be leaving money on the table if we stayed single! Waving the money and the honeymoon under our noses was convincing. We set a date. September 28, 2019. I had four months to pull it together. Meanwhile, visions of homemade pasta and Renaissance frescoes danced in my head.

7. When I told our minister, Rev. Jeff Anderson, about our plans he smiled. Then he said, "As long as you're happy, Eleanor, I approve. Are you happy?" I paused. I said, "I'm

happy enough. Besides, how bad can it be? It's not going to last that long." I meant that one of us would likely die within the next fifteen years. I never contemplated divorce. I figured I could hack it for another decade or so.

8. Greta doesn't like talking about my estate plan, trust, and medical power of attorney. How can I blame her? Maya died when Greta was eleven years old. Ten years later, her half-brother Mark died in a fall down a set of interior stairs in a San Francisco apartment building after a party. Greta got the call at four in the morning and had to drive to the city from Santa Cruz where she was attending college to identify his body. When she called me at five o'clock, she was en route with her new boyfriend Jim. I asked her to put him on the line. "She is all I have," I said. "I need you to promise that you'll take care of her." He responded in a husky voice, "Don't worry. I will." Right then I knew he was the one. Jim stood by Greta in the worst hours of her life.

9. People still talk about Greta and Jim's wedding. They say it was the most beautiful, best-planned wedding they ever attended. It was held on June 23, 2007, at the Regency Center in San Francisco, five years to the day after their first kiss. That day, as I gave my daughter away, I knew that she had accomplished something I never had: a happy, loving relationship that would last. I was so proud I felt filled with helium as I floated through the wedding. Ever since then, I had wanted that happiness, that romantic wedding. I had wanted to stand there like Greta did next to a man I loved and vow until forever.

10. When he came back into my life, Lars vowed never to leave me. But he never vowed to show up in our relationship.

CHAPTER 20
THE WEDDING

I lazed in bed the morning of the wedding, trying to stretch time like an elastic band. But at 8:10, it snapped me across the cheek. I bounded up from a tangle of sheets, frantic.

I had to do my hair, and my makeup, and pick up snacks for the wedding party. A nutritious breakfast. A suite of undergarments to wriggle into—Spanx to cinch the belly—after two kids and four decades, control is a must. Otherwise, I'd never fit into my dress.

By nine o'clock, I was practicing deep belly breathing. I had on sweats and a T-shirt. I didn't want to put on the Spanx till the last minute. I had shampooed my hair and was now frantically drying it. I told myself to inhale, inhale again. Hoist the dryer to the right angle, try not to yank, and ignore the ache in my shoulder as I aimed the nozzle at my sectioned-off hair.

"Patience, girlfriend, patience," I chanted under my breath. "Here I am, at 71, about to be a bride," I said aloud to my reflection. Then I thought, do I even qualify for that title at my advanced age?

I poured myself into a crème-colored silk Nicole Miller sheath with a three-foot train that fit like a glove after six weeks of alterations. We were gathered in an upstairs room of the social hall of my church, surrounded by a full-length mirror, a second-hand couch, and a few chairs.

My girlfriends fussed over me. Greta snapped photos. We ate turkey sandwiches to stave off hunger because the wedding was not until two o'clock.

My youngest granddaughter Amelia bounced around me. "You look beautiful, Mimi!"

Inside the church, she and her sister tossed silk rose petals as I linked arms with Greta and Jim and processed down the aisle. I was in an altered state, so high I felt as if I was floating. Lars beamed like Baldur, the Nordic god of beauty. If I had been a Nordic goddess maybe I would have been Elli, the goddess of old age. A beautiful crone.

As we joined hands at the altar, I felt Lars's solid presence. I snapped back to being mortal. Light from a massive stained-glass window streamed down on us.

He stood there ramrod straight in his navy-blue suit and a teal tie, our wedding colors. I had gone with him to Nordstrom to pick them out. Nordstrom had no teal ties. I was flabbergasted. But Lars was not deterred.

"Let's go look at Nieman Marcus," he suggested.

"You mean Needless Markup?"

I laughed, but I was glad. Not every man would shop several fancy department stores for a tie that matched a wedding color scheme.

Dressed in his finery, he looked distinguished and Scandinavian, his stolid self, but somehow more open and childlike.

He was wide-eyed with excitement as if he were setting off on a great expedition. His voice boomed when he said, "I will," holding both my hands and looking straight at me, something I wished he would do more often.

At that moment he moved me, and tears lapped the corners of my eyes. But I couldn't stop myself from smiling so that my face was a split screen, a comedy tragedy mask, a woman on the verge of committing to forever, however long that might turn out to be.

"I will," he said. Not "I do."

He squeezed my hands so hard I winced, but remembering the sacred moment, the vows, I smiled too.

My turn came. "I will," I said, my voice corn-silk and husk, muted, yet strong.

When the minister got to "until death do us part" and I had to repeat the phrase, my voice caught for what seemed an everlasting moment.

Time is like silly putty, I thought. Not a rubber band. It is infinitely flexible, you can stretch and bend it, or ball it up and bounce it down the stairs. Then the minister said some lovely Rumi-like poetic words and I snapped back into the moment.

"There are a thousand ways to kneel and kiss the ground," or something similar.

All is holy, I thought, even the pinching undergarments, the way the train of my dress fell in a river behind me, how Lars's cheeks looked like a happy squirrel's stuffed with nuts, about to bury his treasure.

I want to be married, I thought. *But I don't want to be a wife.*

I felt sun blinded, stunned by my thoughts as if I might fall over. But Lars held my hands, held me tight, my palms beginning to feel like melting icing. Suddenly, I wanted to pull back, to say "I won't." I won't be anyone's wife.

I'm a bride wearing white silk, carrying a white bouquet, I thought. I can't be that woman bent over the kitchen sink, scouring, hanging laundry on a cracked plastic rack, or bringing my overly optimistic husband with his squirrel cheeks down to earth. Not that!

The minister introduced us as "Eleanor and Lars, newly married partners." We turned and Lars held my hand up to help me down the stairs from the altar. Our friends and family stood and applauded. Again, the feeling of floating as we glided down the aisle. We went into the office at the back of the sanctuary, and magically, glasses of champagne appeared.

The wedding party cracked jokes. We signed the marriage certificate and then went outside to take photos. Later, in the social hall, we danced to Zydeco tunes and 1960s oldies, listened to toasts, and of course, cut the cake. Our conglomeration of friends and family—writers, artists, and other eccentrics on my side, and Kiwanis and business connections for Lars—all played well together, and the wine and appetizers vanished before we got any.

There's a photo of five-year-old Amelia, her sister Zoe, and their friends lying in the middle of the wooden dance floor in a circle, their heads touching like the center of a daisy, their bodies radiating into the room like petals. Another favorite photo: a closeup of my friend Navneet holding one of the little green plants we gave as wedding favors, the terra cotta pot orange against her brown hands, the succulent unfolding like a series of blooming hearts.

We held a dinner in the courtyard of a local hotel for a smaller group of family and friends. Later, after a final round of toasts at the bar, we retired to our room, a "petite suite" with a sitting area and a king-size bed.

We were in high spirits, mildly drunk, and emotionally exhausted. We fell asleep without making love. An hour later I woke up with a sense that something was missing. I leaned over and gently jostled my new husband's warm shoulder. He mumbled, then turned to face me.

I whispered, "Don't you think we need to make love?"

Lars stirred, finally awoke fully, and began caressing me. Then he said a Norwegian phrase he had taught me, "*jeg elsker deg.*"

To my ear, it sounded like *ya ilska dai.* It means "I love you."

"Wait, say that again," I pleaded, my eyes unfocused in the dark bedroom. I snuggled against Lars's chest, inhaling the essential oil he used, Night Rain, from The Body Shop on Telegraph Avenue. It was musky, slightly overpowering, but combined with his natural scent more like a forest of pine trees.

"*Jeg elsker deg,*" he repeated.

I said it back to him.

"Not bad," he said. "But it's pronounced like 'dye' not 'day.'"

I said it back to him in the same sing-song rhythm. I liked it, like a little song, *jeg elsker deg, jeg elsker deg.* Sort of like "Daisy, Daisy Give me Your Answer Do," one of my favorite childhood ditties. It was easy to get lost in the language. Lars rarely told me he loved me in English, so this was special.

There's a photo of Lars as a toddler before his parents emigrated. He's dressed in a white cotton T-shirt and a pair of woolen rompers held up with straps. He's holding a furry toy, but I can't tell if it's a bear. He has blonde curls that poof over his forehead and a smile that seems to say, "Oh, all right, if I must," but his eyes look like he's about to cry. He came to the United States when he was not yet two, but old enough to understand *jeg elsker deg*.

With Lars, it was hard to tell if he was making love because he enjoyed it, or only because it pleased me. He was usually eerily silent, and I only knew he was about to orgasm because he began to move more urgently. That night, though, after I'd come several times, he burrowed into me fiercely, and just before he came, I heard that sing-song phrase again, nestled inside my newlywed mind.

"I love you," I said, in short gasps.

"I love you too," he said back.

The next morning, I awoke to the gurgle of the Keurig machine and the smell of espresso. I pushed up on one elbow. Lars stood naked in front of the highboy under an antique map of Paris in a gilt frame brewing the coffee. The hotel had real creamer, and he brought me a coffee the color of caramel, and a slice of wedding cake on a small plate.

Nothing before or since has ever tasted as sweet.

He climbed back in bed and watched as I sipped my coffee and ate my cake, pausing to give him bites, and sighing again over how delicious it was.

"We did it," he said.

"We sure did," I said.

Later, after we dressed, we met my brother and his wife and Greta and Jim and the girls for breakfast, a sumptuous brunch complete with smoked salmon, made-to-order omelets, fresh fruit, and French pastries. We glided through the day wrapped in the afterglow of our very romantic wedding. Every so often, I repeated to myself, *jeg elsker deg*, and then said it to Lars.

Two days later we were on a plane to Pisa, Italy. Our driver got lost on the way to our hotel in Riomaggiore, the first of the towns in the Cinque Terre, and let us out in the town square. We had to drag our luggage up a steep hill to reach the hotel. We fell into bed exhausted. When I opened my eyes the next morning, I snuggled into my husband and said *ti amo*, instead.

After our glorious Italian sojourn, we visited Basel, Switzerland where I had spent my junior year in college living with a Swiss family, the Metzgers. This was my fifth visit. Any time I went to Europe, Basel was on the itinerary. To say I was close with this family is an understatement—they showed me what a happy, functional family was, and included me in it.

My host father Martin Metzger was patient with my American ways. Over time, he became the closest thing to a real father I had ever known. He was protective of me as a risk-taking twenty-year-old and warned me against dating men I met casually in parks or at parties. I did not always heed his advice, but I revered him.

When Lars sat on the sofa next to Martin (now in his nineties and profoundly deaf) and talked to him about politics, patiently repeating himself, Martin not only responded, a rarity with strangers, but he grinned. They had a spirited discussion. I was beside myself with happiness. My new husband and my adopted father hit it off. This seemed like a vital stamp of approval.

Lars had charmed everyone.

As our plane lifted above Zurich and then soared parallel to the Alps, I leaned into the window well and snapped photos. The sun backlit the mountains. We banked toward the West and my body tilted against Lars. He squeezed my thigh. I glowed, immersed in happiness. I had no idea how the next months would unfold.

PART III
TOGETHER APART

CHAPTER 21
WHAT HONEYMOON?

I stood in our kitchen quivering. My left eye twitched. I wanted to shout at Lars, *I'm out of here! Our marriage is a charade!* I gulped down angry words in hot chunks.

Not even a year in, and we were teetering on the hairy edge.

I stared at my husband, eyes blazing. He had just exploded when I asked if he wanted to go out and join a neighborhood singalong. He growled at me and clenched his teeth.

What is wrong with you? The question lingered in a thought bubble above my head, but I didn't think this was the opportune moment to speak.

He puffed his cheeks and blew out, a long whoosh of held breath.

I remembered a moment years ago on the dance floor. It was a Friday night at Eagles, and I'd danced so much I could feel the blood pounding in my cheeks. Heat rose from my chest to my face in waves. We were slow dancing, and suddenly Lars leaned in. I thought he was going to whisper something to me. Instead, I felt the slightest breeze against my skin. It sent shivers up my spine. Lars was blowing on my neck. I reared back and looked at him. We'd been dance partners for only a few weeks. It was a bold move from a man who was bookish, courtly, and seemingly reserved.

Up until then, I thought he was standoffish, not interested me romantically. As his breath cooled my overheated skin, I felt gobsmacked. Pleased. Nervous in the best way.

Now, we faced off in front of the stove, the house suddenly so silent I could hear the refrigerator hum. Lars gazed out the window. I stayed riveted on his face. What made leaving our marriage unimaginable was the improbability of it ever happening in the first place. What were the odds? A million to one, I figured. Yet here we were, supposedly newlyweds, locked in combat only months after our blissful honeymoon.

"I need a break," I said. I had to get out of the house. Now.

I'd been here too many times. With other men. In other relationships. A point of exasperation where I snapped and hasty words tumbled out. And then either I left, or the man did. I flashed back to that street corner in Palma, and Saeed's stricken face when I yelled at him. I was tired of repeating my old patterns.

Not this time, I told myself.

I went to the front hallway. I grabbed my purse and my car keys. I shut the front door softly to shield Lars from my fury.

I punched the garage keypad, the door rolled up. I was in the car and out onto the street before I asked myself where I was going.

"You're running away from home," I said aloud.

We'd been married for just eight months, and I wasn't sure if we'd stay together long enough to celebrate our first anniversary.

A happy memory two days after our wedding, we woke up in a small hotel high above the harbor in the hill town of Riomaggiore, immersed in *la dolce vita.* Each morning the innkeeper brought us frothy cappuccinos and pastries in the tiny breakfast room as we talked about which new adventure we would try that day. We ambled along a short section of the Via dell'Amore, a spectacular path that leads to Manarola, another of the Cinque Terre hill towns, hypnotized by rolling waves crashing against the cliffs. We visited a local vineyard on a terraced hillside where the grapes were transported by boat to be made into private-label white wine. We took a romantic boat trip to Porto Venere.

When we returned home to Walnut Creek, my photo stream was filled with pictures of the Ligurian Sea, selfies of the two of us shoulder to shoulder at café tables, and photos of pasta drenched in pesto with a sweating bottle of wine in the background. We lived immersed in a haze of blue sky and undulating water. We came back to a dusty, fire-smudged Northern California.

I lived suspended in Italian bliss for several days, slowly, painfully getting home for real: cleaning the refrigerator, sorting through a box of unopened mail, deleting emails, until the blue sea and sky had faded into shortening days and even longer nights.

A bucket of ice-cold water hit me in the face in early December, six weeks after we got home. One morning after we made love, I began to bleed. At first, soaking thin "light days" pads with rusty spots, and then suddenly a clot. My vagina felt heavy and raw. I made an appointment. Suddenly I found myself in a starchy gown with my feet in stirrups, staring through the V-shape of my parted knees at my gynecologist.

I was years past menopause, and I'd had a partial hysterectomy when I was in my mid-forties, so bleeding was alarming. Where was it coming from, and why?

My doctor had called her medical assistant into the room, and I could hear them rustling, arranging things, preparing. Metal clinked and I could hear a sound like ripping paper. I stared at the pierced holes in the ceiling tile, little black pinpricks, a random galaxy spread above me. My heels in the stirrups were cold, the metal hard and unforgiving. I put my hands on my belly under the drape and breathed slowly, puffing out my cheeks in a Lamaze breath.

"Relax," I told myself, "It's going to be okay," but my inner voice didn't sound entirely sincere, as in, "Yeah sure it will be okay when it's *over*."

The medical assistant came and stood next to me. My doctor said I'd feel pressure. She had picked up an instrument, turned away from the metal tray, and perched on the stool at the foot of the table between my legs.

"Take a deep breath, Eleanor," she said and just as the bottom third of my lungs filled, she jabbed me with something much bigger and much sharper than I had anticipated.

"Help!" I said, and then again more softly, "Help, help!"

"Are you saying 'help'?"

"Yes," I said. I squeezed the medical assistant's hand as hard as I could and huffed my big Lamaze breath. I wanted to say, *Fuck, yes, I'm saying help. You just stabbed me!*

My doctor said she'd have results back in about a week and meantime not to worry it's probably nothing. The medical assistant handed me a paper towel and a few wet wipes to clean myself and closed the door softly. I opened the wipes and touched my throbbing vulva as gently as I could. I'd probably have more bleeding, the doctor had said, so I opened the sanitary napkin they left for me in its oblong box and pasted it in my panties.

I felt numb as an iceberg by the time I made it to the elevator. When I went out through the sliding glass doors, the winter sunlight held my face like two hands on either side of my cheeks, making my eyes blink. I was so happy to be outside! I walked to my car like a normal person, in my every day, trying not to think too hard about what had just happened. I thought it was going to be a PAP smear. Instead, I'd had a biopsy.

At home, I put a heating pad on my belly. I asked Lars to bring me ibuprofen. I hadn't had cramps this painful in more than twenty-five years, since before my partial hysterectomy. I snuggled under a Pendleton blanket in our living room, the wool scratchy and warm, the blanket heavy, holding me in the chair each time a new wave of cramps swamped me.

A week later I got the diagnosis: a rare, aggressive cervical cancer called clear cell carcinoma. Typically, this kind of cancer affects the kidneys. How did it form in my cervix? No one knew, but it was not the usual cervical cancer caused by HPV.

My doctor fast-tracked a referral to a cancer specialist. In the week between diagnosis and consultation, I asked Lars to promise that if I died, he'd continue to have our housekeeper clean every other week. If he let the house go rogue, I said I would haunt him.

"You're going to haunt me anyway," he said.

On Christmas Eve, we met with a surgeon. Sitting in his office that Tuesday, I watched intently as he pointed out pictures of reproductive organs on his giant computer screen. I felt oddly comforted. He offered science. And hope—we'd found this early. With quick action, I might be among the lucky few to escape chemo and radiation, the fear and mess of recurrences, and the side effects of treatment.

In the second week of January, I had surgery to remove my remaining reproductive organs: my cervix, ovaries, and fallopian tubes. I surrendered my body to modern medicine and with help from a cocktail of drugs, I sank into oblivion.

The first thing I remembered after the operation was hearing my husband's laughter. He and the male recovery room nurse were telling guy jokes. Lost in the fog of anesthesia, I paddled furiously to the surface, breathing with effort.

"Hello," I said. My brain felt gummy.

"Hi, hon," Lars said. "How are you feeling?"

"So glad it's over," I croaked.

The pathology results came back a week later: Stage 1. No spread. No further treatment. I'd be under surveillance for the next five years; I was a cancer survivor.

Lars had been a brick during the ordeal, reassuring me that we were in this together, that I didn't have to face it alone. The night of my diagnosis I had walked around my living room chanting the mantra attributed to John Lennon: "Life is what happens when you're busy making other plans."

Cancer was not in my plans. Lars and I were newlyweds, not yet three months married. I never expected our vows to be tested so soon. Until that night, I was protected by the hypnotic hubris of mortals when confronted with death: denial. If Lars and I hadn't made love early in December, if I hadn't bled afterward, those cancer cells would have continued to multiply deep in my belly. I would not have known.

Accident? Luck? Divine intervention? Who knows? And does it matter, in the end, how miracles occur? Just as I began to trust that I was going to live after all, another unexpected monster jumped out of its hole. But this time, it affected everyone.

CHAPTER 22
LOCKED DOWN

We lived tucked away in a valley on the outskirts, far from the streets of San Francisco or Oakland. Our village of 10,000 elders went into seclusion even before the Bay Area counties issued "shelter in place" orders in mid-March of 2020. Red circles of COVID-19 outbreaks widened and merged on the John Hopkins tracking app. We were old and thus vulnerable.

Walking on the empty golf course, I saw a fawn toddling on spindly legs behind its mother. The doe turned and looked at me and I thought, "I don't have to stay away from you."

When I saw a hummingbird hovering, I moved next to it, whispering, cajoling. It dipped its beak deep into the flower's heart and kept on feeding, unafraid.

Humans were more skittish, and with reason. Everyone at Rossmoor was in the high-risk group. When Lars and I encountered neighbors on our walks, we'd step off the paths and onto the manicured grass. I was still recovering from surgery, just beginning to feel well enough to go for longer walks.

Proper social distancing became an art form, one we embellished with calls of "How are you?" and "Beautiful day!"

In the 1950s, polio was the scourge. We sucked on sugar cubes infused with the vaccine, and now people hardly remembered iron lungs. We needed scientists to develop a vaccine for COVID-19 and labs to manufacture tons of it, but we also needed wild turkeys, robins, and deer to hold us up until solitary confinement was over.

Lars spent hours reading on his iPad, his face enclosed in a digital fishbowl, reflecting the screen glow. I couldn't break through unless I went over and touched his shoulder. He'd look up slowly, like a turtle poking its head out of its shell, exploring the world he'd left behind, the too-noisy, too-bright world, the one where I existed.

Come back, my love, I need you, I wanted to say. Yet I didn't speak.

I felt exposed and vulnerable. Hemmed in by our constant togetherness.

One Saturday I was watching a concert on TV, stretched out in the Relax-the-Back chair, entranced by the flight of the pianist's fingers over the keyboard.

I called to Lars. He was in his office, checking email, I assumed.

"Honey, you have to see this," I yelled.

A few minutes later I called again, "This is amazing. Come see!"

At last, I hauled myself out of the chair and went to stand in his office doorway.

"Come look at this pianist," I urged.

Lars quarter-turned so I was in his peripheral vision. Then he slammed both hands on his desk with a bang. His keyboard shimmied. Papers rustled to the floor. I jumped.

"Will you leave me alone?" he shouted. "Can't you see I'm busy?!"

I trembled from his lightning flash of rage, an emotion he rarely displayed.

I backed into the hallway. He had bi-fold doors in his office. Instinctively, I grabbed them by the handles and attempted to slam them shut. Slamming a bifold door is impossible—the bottom dragged over the carpet. There was no doorframe to bang against. The doors closed with a pathetic whimper, then immediately gapped open.

I turned in a huff, realizing how ridiculous I must have looked, and burst out laughing at my fool self. I spent the afternoon alone, alternately brooding and watching home remodeling shows on HGTV. At least some things could be fixed.

One minute I'd feel calm and grounded, the next I'd be over the moon with anxiety—and the triggers were everywhere—from my iPhone to the radio and TV, to my husband.

Lars insisted he was following prevention guidelines, and perhaps he was, but I saw scant evidence of this. He appeared to go hours without washing his hands, and when he did it was a nonchalant effort. Was he singing two choruses of "Happy Birthday"? Was he using hot water? He put the recycling in the outside shared bin and didn't use sanitizer or wash afterward.

He was an adult capable of making his own decisions, I told myself, but his casual approach might have ended up killing us or at least making us seriously ill. I lived in terror of his getting infected with the virus and becoming his caregiver, which meant I'd get COVID-19 too.

To me. he appeared to behave like an overgrown child. Defiant. Rebellious. He refused to drink water, something experts advised in the best of times; during COVID, it was vital to stay hydrated to try to thin mucus secretions. When I tried to explain that to him, he stared at me like I was from another planet.

I had built my sense of security on mothering others beginning as a three-year-old when my mother was too depressed to care for me and my younger sister and brother. I had to fight ingrained habits. I kept reminding myself, *"I'm not his mother!"*

Lars exerted control over objects, not people. He began working on a 1000-piece jigsaw puzzle of—wait for it—pencils! There was no discernable pattern or pretty landscape.

Just row after row of yellow number 2 pencils.

He set up a card table with puzzle pieces laid out in neat rows, a second table where he kept partially assembled pieces, and a third table with the puzzle on it. It was a brilliant strategy. Every time I looked at it, I went cross-eyed.

Between bouts of reading on his iPad or assembling the pencils, he was at his command station in his office with three giant computer monitors working remotely.

Computers were his comfort zone. They are logical. People are not.

Strong feelings of any kind, particularly his own, made him freeze. In conversation, he would usually change the subject to something intellectual, arcane, and even bizarre. His mind was active and curious, which I loved, but sometimes I'd get an overwhelming urge to make him stop talking about strange theories, obscure authors, or irrelevant details. I'd sit on my hands, clamp my lips together, and let him ramble. It was torture.

I loved him. And he drove me crazy. I realized we'd likely be sequestered in our house together for several months. Little did I know!

⬧

My husband's voice boomed through the house, hearty as a bowl of porridge. He projected Papa Bear qualities, jolly as can be with clients or business associates. He was a head and a half taller than me, and when we walked outside holding hands, he matched his steps to mine and shouted cheery greetings to neighbors.

The difference between his outside persona, and the self he showed me in private was stark. Did he have multiple personalities? I began to wonder whether he was the same man I thought I had married, my gallant dance partner, now grown rigid and cold.

"I canceled the hotels today," I told him on one of our walks. "United Airlines is giving me a credit for the flight, but we have to use it by the end of 2021."

Before the pandemic that would have seemed like a huge window of time. Now it seemed like not enough. Our trip to Hawaii was off. The future was foreshortened. Projecting beyond the next day seemed crazily optimistic.

"Will we ever travel again?" I asked.

"Of course," he said in his Papa Bear voice.

If I tried to look into the future, I saw catastrophe or some gauzy storybook outcome. Neither was real. Only the everlasting, ever-loving NOW was.

⬧

"The Kumbaya moment has passed," a fellow writer said during a video chat.

I thought, *That can't be right.* At that point, a few weeks into the Bay Area's shelter-in-place order, I was still sticking to a daily schedule, checking in with my writing community on Slack every morning, putting virtual literary events in my calendar, baking muffins, attending daily meditation sessions with my Sangha on Zoom—all the "productive" things that were holding my depression and freak out at bay.

Three months into this interminable purgatory, I was circling the lake of fire imagining that eventually, if I was careful and good, I'd make it past COVID alive. Social isolation took a toll. That and having my husband of eight months in the house 24/7 on computer support calls, offering loud advice, and holding jolly cocktail hours with his Kiwanis group on Zoom three nights a week.

Slowly, slowly I was going mad.

The Kumbaya moment *was* over. It evaporated along with the uplifting quotes, hopeful poems, and stories about a brand-new society where everyone would wear Earth shoes and drive electric cars. They flitted across social media feeds like crepe paper streamers.

One member of my writing group said on a Zoom call: "I've had my life. I don't care if I get COVID. That worry is for younger people." I wanted to stand up like Steve Martin with a fake arrow through my head and yell, "Well, excussseeee me."

I wanted every single precious moment of my life. Just because I'd lived a long time, that didn't mean I wanted it to be over. Cancer had locked in my commitment to go on living. But I had one overriding question. How would Lars and I find a way to stay in step?

By August, despair had become an anchor. We hadn't had sex in three months. I was hungry for intimacy, for a tender word, or glance, or touch. We hugged each morning, but it was like hugging a brother, not a lover.

I tried to talk to him. I focused on "I" statement"—how lonely I felt, how not having any sex life had become so painful that I'd started avoiding thinking or talking about sex.

At one point I asked him flat out, "Is our sex life over? If it is, I'd at least like to know..."

"I don't have an answer for you," he said, holding my hand in the dark bedroom, the two of us like wooden dolls lying side by side in our big bed.

"Is there someone else?" I asked.

He laughed and said no.

"You laugh," I said, "but I can't find any explanations."

I picked up a book on neurodiverse relationships and read this: "If you are doing the work for two, you will get tired, stressed, and eventually, you will burn out. You need to know that you are not the only one keeping the relationship together."

But what I knew was the opposite. Lars had checked out. I didn't know how to get him to re-engage, or even if it would be possible. The next day I called and made an appointment with another couple's therapist.

CHAPTER 23
MORE STUFF I LEFT OUT

1. I never planned on getting married late in life. I wanted a loving relationship—a committed partner—but marriage? At my age? I'd lived alone, sometimes with a partner, sometimes without, for thirty-five years. I'd raised two daughters from two brief marriages. Had a career. Bought and sold three houses. Managed my own money. Traveled by myself. I was lonely, yes, sometimes to the point of despair, but I always bounced back to acceptance of who I was, my limitations, my strengths, and what I thought of as my interesting but challenging personality. I thought—with good evidence—that I was too independent, too strong-minded for most men my age. I wanted love, but not necessarily "until death do us part."

2. When Lars came along and texted me a new Japanese haiku each morning, when he opened doors and carried boxes and bags, and when he kissed my hand after each dance, I began to doubt my resolve to stay single. He charmed me with gallantry and reeled me in with his quirky intelligence. I was drawn to his iconoclastic personality, his penchant for expensive hats, his passion for theater and

movies, and his obsessive reading habits. He was not like other men I had dated. When I discovered what a skillful and considerate lover he was, I was hooked.

3. It wasn't until after we married that I understood how hard Lars had worked to woo me; how much "autistic masking" he was doing to act as if he was neurotypical; and how difficult, if not impossible, it would be for him to sustain intimacy over time. Author Maxine Aston describes this aspect of the ASD male this way: "Often in the beginning of [the] relationship, the female partner may have felt she was the center of his attention and been very flattered by the devotion and consideration he showed her. He will have made her feel very special and in some cases flooded her with gifts and romantic gestures. This passionate initial stage can end quite quickly and once they marry or live together it can come to a rather abrupt end; she will be left wondering what went wrong, or worse still, what she did wrong." When I read this passage, a light bulb went on. I realized that in those early months of courtship, Lars had been acting as if he knew how to be an intimate partner. He was skillful at masking his autism, and that was likely exhausting him just as he was reeling me in. I had wanted to be courted. He had seemed so considerate, so enthusiastic, so devoted to pleasing me.

4. Sometimes memories burst over me like a water-filled balloon. Suddenly, it's 1954 and I'm back in Miss Crow's first-grade class about to march in the Thanksgiving parade. Some children are cowboys, some are Indians, the only descriptors we knew at the time. The cowboys are dressed in fringed vests like the ones Karen and Kenny

wear on Mickey Mouse Club, with cap pistols in holsters. Even real cowboy hats and boots! My mother would never buy clothes like that, so I'm an Indian dressed in a brown paper tunic I cut out myself with blunt scissors from grocery bags, then stapled together, coloring feathers to paste onto a paper headdress that wobbles and threatens to pull apart when I put it on. Were there cowboys at the first Thanksgiving? Even at six, I know better, because Mom reads us stories: Laura Ingalls Wilder, the Greek myths, and tales of Celtic warrior women. Cowboys were out West, and there was no out West at the first Thanksgiving. Red-faced, squirming in my paper sack dress, I lined up behind the cowboys. We marched out to the asphalt playground. So many things are wrong.

5. For my high school graduation, my grandmother gave me a set of Samsonite luggage. It was textured beige and it looked like fake alligator hide. It had silver clasps and a faux alligator skin handle. I'd never had my own luggage before and this four-piece set made me feel like one of the models in my grandmother's Vogue magazines, or like a Hyannis Port socialite like Jackie Kennedy. I even had a drop waist lamb's wool coat, also a gift from grandma, to carry out my imaginary glamorous life. But the luggage! That was a whole new level. The biggest suitcase gaped like an open mouth, its two sides lined with green quilted padding, each side with a separate lid that could be latched once the contents were packed.

6. I carefully considered what to pack and what to leave behind for my trip to college. I pictured myself unpacking what I hadn't yet packed. When you're young, you imagine that other people live much like your own family.

Of course, I knew this couldn't be true. I'd read plenty of novels with settings from ships at sea to English drawing rooms to meat packing plants in the Midwest, but I still didn't quite get how very differently people lived from one home to the next. I paced in front of the open suitcase. Would my roommates wear jeans? Would they have nice clothes? I'd worked as a salesgirl at the Red Robin boutique on 185th Street, and at the downtown Halle's department store to make extra money. I bought my own clothes. I was determined never to dress in the equivalent of a brown paper sack tunic again as long as I lived!

7. Dressed in my wedding finery I was about as far from a brown paper tunic as a girl could get. That silk Nicole Miller gown (purchased at a bargain price from a wedding store that specialized in discontinued designer dresses) was the anti-paper sack outfit. Grandma would have approved; Mom would have been horrified since she typically dressed in men's overalls and work shirts and repeatedly told me that I was too vain. I also wore an antique lace three-quarter-length sleeve bolero jacket, adding a touch of sophisticated modesty to the ensemble. Originally, the dress was strapless, but during alterations, I decided to add straps. I didn't want to spend my wedding day tugging up the bodice of my dress. It offended my sense of propriety, of having graduated with my fancy luggage.

8. Because of our ages, Lars and I had no biological parents at our wedding. But we did have spiritual parents, mentors who had helped us close the gaps in our emotional upbringing. Given our ages, some of our mentors were elderly. Lars had a friend from Kiwanis who had long

urged him to find domestic bliss. Dave's fondest wish was for Lars to be married, settled, and looked after. Dave and his wife Susan sat in the front row on Lars's side of the church. I liked Dave, although I didn't know him well. He was wheelchair-bound and had a caregiver at his side at the reception. I leaned over, and hugged him, careful not to slosh my glass of champagne. He beamed.

9. Later, he told Lars that our wedding had been one of the happiest occasions of his life.

10. At the San Francisco airport waiting for the plane to take us to Italy two days later we got a call from a mutual friend, another of Lars's mentors. He said he was calling with sad news. Moments after Dave left our reception, he had a massive stroke. Susan and the caregiver managed to get him in the car, but he had lost consciousness. They drove him to the hospital. There he lingered for some hours but was ultimately pronounced dead. We were stunned. Lars said, "At least I made him happy at the end."

CHAPTER 24
TWO FISH

"I got my layoff notice," Lars said. He gazed at the food on his plate. "They are firing thirteen people because of the pandemic. I'm getting two weeks' severance pay."

I reached across our dining room table and squeezed his hand. I thought he might cry.

"They are using COVID as an excuse to unload their highly paid employees," I said.

Age discrimination made me furious. I called an employment lawyer in the city I knew to help get him a better settlement. Lars had worked for his company as a consultant for more than twenty-five years and then transitioned to being an employee three years earlier. We relied on his income. We scrambled to rejigger our budget and ensure we could pay our mortgage.

Our days blurred together in a haze of wildfire smoke, double masking to go buy groceries, CDC advisories, Zoom calls, and financial upheaval. We briefly considered leaving Rossmoor but neither of us could picture selling the house we'd so recently bought. A major move would only double our grief.

While he was an employee, Lars had kept his other consulting clients, working nights and weekends on their projects. He doubled down, calling or emailing in search of more work. I increased the amounts I drew from my retirement funds. We cut back on eating out and canceled travel plans.

The post-honeymoon year was only half over. Already another crisis.

☐

We had stopped going to Zydeco dances, another casualty of the pandemic. Unless we were outside, socializing was taboo, and dancing in groups was out of the question. I could barely remember our life in the "before time" when we connected through dancing, socializing, and cultural events. We drifted farther apart, almost imperceptibly, yet I could sense it in the way we had begun to avoid even talking about having sex.

Lars hadn't touched me in any way that felt tender in months.

One morning I awoke before dawn. I was so sexually frustrated that my vulva ached. I pulled myself up on one elbow and stared at my sleeping husband. We hadn't made love in so long I had forgotten how. In our old life, I thought a few weeks was a long time. Now, it seemed like child's play. I had a sudden urge to punch Lars in the head, just haul off and clobber him. I shook with suppressed fury.

"What is the matter with us?" I spoke out loud into the empty air.

Marlowe was lying on the pillow just above Lars's head, and he stirred, one green eye blinking open. I knew I'd never get an answer from my husband. I tossed off the covers and stalked out of the bedroom.

☐

I confessed to friends that my marriage hung by a thread, and that I suspected that Lars was autistic. I described how he shut me out. A wall had grown up between us.

A common refrain became: "That's just a guy thing. All men are like that."

I'd get some version of, "Just deal with it!"

The advice was well-meaning. All marriages have issues, many men are clueless about feelings, and women have to do the bulk of the emotional labor. But that presumes the man in question is simply unaware of his feelings. Neurodivergent men are different. Feelings for them are like the mysteries of the universe, giant black holes, galactic nothingness.

Lars was not just a clueless guy drinking beer and watching the 49ers game on Sunday afternoons ignoring his wife. He was brilliant about things he was interested in, namely technology, science, philosophy, and art. He also happened to hate TV sports, and sports in general, although he was very gifted with a croquet mallet or on the bocce ball court.

When I reported his neglect and rudeness, his complete coldness, and what I got back was, "That's just what guys do" I wanted to scream, "NO IT IS NOT!"

I was on a steep learning curve. I was being coached in therapy and support groups for non-autistic spouses to actively manage myself: Avoid eye contact or confrontation, when possible. Curtail my feelings or parse them carefully. Don't overwhelm him with emotions or demands. I was crocheting a giant ball of avoided feelings.

There is a Greek word for the inability to process or express emotion, "Alexithymia." The literal meaning is "no words for feelings."

"Research has now shown that being in a relationship with a partner with Alexithymia will negatively affect relationship satisfaction and quality," I read in one of the autism books I poured over, looking for answers.

I tried to make sense of what was happening to me. It was weird. I had begun to lose track of who I was as a person. Our marriage had turned into a game of emotional Whack-a-Mole or as our therapist put it, "A cycle of unresolved conflict."

Inside his wedding band, Lars had the phrase "Okay then, 2018" inscribed in small gold letters. It used to be our little joke. How our courtship year unfolded like the snap of a flamenco dancer's fan—fast, bright, and sassy.

Now, I wished we could roll back the clock to a time that was more than infatuation but less than marital lockdown. I had naively believed that I could handle our differences, that somehow loving Lars had given me magical powers. I think he naively believed he could go on masking, that he could pretend to tolerate our mismatch.

One by one, clues about our opposite neurotypes piled up. Even the way we dressed.

Lars wore a crisp permanent press button-down shirt, always long-sleeved, no matter the weather, along with black Dockers jeans. In summer, a straw fedora, in winter a felted one, sometimes with a small jaunty feather. When we were falling in love, I had noticed how crisp his shirts were, how they held the smell of detergent in the collars.

Over time, I understood how his uniform served him. Easy to launder, it didn't require ironing and perfectly matched his no-nonsense, literal personality. It offered a brilliant answer to the question of what to wear day after day, year after year.

While Lars kept things simple, I over-complicated them. My closet was filled with fussy silk and rayon, in bright colors, clothes that required special care and handling.

Much as I tried, I lost patience. I yelled or threatened to leave. I forgot about "I" statements.

When I could remember who we had been to each other in 2018, I could still imagine Lars holding me on the dance floor, his hand guiding me, the agile way he moved to the music.

"Maybe I'm just a selfish bastard," Lars said.

We were on my laptop, talking with our therapist Jonathan on Zoom.

I turned toward Lars. "No, honey, it's just that your brain is wired differently."

I reached over and patted his arm.

Jonathan made an artfully phrased observation about the "inner critic" and reminded Lars that in a marriage both people are responsible for caring for what he referred to as our "puppy." This marriage we'd entered was like adopting a puppy that we both needed to love. There were three entities present: Lars, Eleanor, and the puppy. We each had needs.

The poor puppy is whimpering in the corner, dehydrated and begging for kibble, I thought, but I bit my lip and went back to coloring mandalas in my *Extreme Stress Mender* workbook with fine point sharpies.

I completed dozens of mandalas during our months of Zoom therapy. I couldn't just sit there during agonizing silences and Lars's long, circuitous, highly intellectualized answers to Jonathan's probing questions. I had to do *something*. Even our therapy was making me insane.

The mismatch between his theorizing and my urgent need to fix our marriage felt like quicksand. The more I struggled, the deeper I sank.

"You *are* a selfish bastard, Lars!"

I lobbed those words like a grenade. It was after he had left me sitting in a downtown restaurant waiting for him. He hadn't responded to my texts or phone calls. I had sat there eating alone, staring into my salad as if it held the answers, humiliated. I was furious.

"I deserve so much better," I said.

I couldn't shake off the humiliation. The way the wait staff looked concerned as the time dragged on. I felt the sting of being brushed off, and a flame of rage surged in my chest.

For the first time, I thought seriously about divorce. I was desperately lonely.

I decided it didn't matter whether Lars was on the autism spectrum or not. We'd never know for sure, anyway, because even after I had found a psychologist who diagnosed adults, my husband said he was too expensive and refused to see him.

Lars was completely absorbed by his own needs, unable to break out of his bubble—"The squirrel cage," as he called it, where he ruminated over and over about some perceived shortcoming of his, or some imagined criticism I'd leveled.

"You *are* a selfish bastard," I repeated, staring straight at him, facing off across the dining room table.

"I'm going to take a page out of your book. I'm going to be a selfish bastard, too," I said, keeping my voice level so that he would pay attention. "I'm going to leave when I need space, hang out with friends, and take care of myself."

"You should," he said, giving me the equivalent of a Papal dispensation.

His eyes flickered with recognition then looked away. It was that *away* that got to me, the darting off, the way the blue of his eyes deepened to gray as he flicked them off to a neutral zone. His face closed like a curtain drawn shut by a fastidious widow. He stared into the middle distance, looking past me. Not blankness as much as willful closure. He hardened his body and made himself absent.

Where are you? I wanted to ask. But in asking, I knew I'd drive him further away.

Our couples' therapist said we were like two fish. I was an ocean fish. Lars was a freshwater fish. But we swam together in the brackish waters where the river meets the sea. When those waters got muddied by our mismatched communications, we lost our way. It was a pretty metaphor, but in the end an unsatisfying one. I couldn't see in the brackish water, I couldn't even breathe, I couldn't be my own kind of fish and still survive.

In the middle of our fight, I realized that I desperately needed oxygen, the open ocean, and the illusion that I could swim away. A friend agreed to loan me her place for a week while she went back East. I packed a bag, took my laptop and my favorite pillow, and left my husband.

CHAPTER 25
HOME

Only two days later I went home to pick up the mail, fix a nutritious meal, and check-in. I told myself I was worried about Lars. But it was really myself I was worried about. And us. After dinner each night I went back and slept at Jane's place, attempting to calm myself. I read. I meditated. I wrote in my journal. I talked to my therapist, Amy. By the end of that week, I missed Lars and Marlowe so much, that I couldn't wait to get home. I came home and we fell into our old routines. By a miracle, we were back together. We had reset, at least for the moment.

CHAPTER 26
SCAR TISSUE

On the other end of the restaurant patio, a few other couples were dining. It was a beautiful spring evening. We sipped our wine and chatted about summer travel plans, my upcoming birthday, Lars's computer and database consulting, and my grandkids. This and that.

The waiter set down my shrimp Louis salad (with dressing on the side) and Lars's grilled Portobello mushroom with polenta (smothered in ricotta cheese and tomato sauce). Just then, my husband's phone chimed. He took the call.

I never answered my phone anytime I was face to face with another human being. But as a tech maven, Lars always answered his phone, no matter what. I focused on the meal in front of me, the glistening baby shrimp, the perfectly cut hard-boiled egg, and the pale green avocado.

Lars's voice boomed, but I didn't listen to the words. I'd learned to block out the details of computer support calls. But when he said, "Hello, Dr. Moon," I tuned in.

Lars had had two prostate-specific antigen or PSA tests, and both came back with elevated levels. On Monday he had his prostate gland biopsied, a very invasive procedure, and refused so much as an aspirin for the discomfort. I was expecting a diagnosis of an enlarged prostate and wondering what the treatment would be.

"So, I have prostate cancer!" His voice boomed across the patio.

Lars smiled as if the doctor had just told him he'd won the lottery. I set down my fork. Suddenly my shrimp and avocado didn't look so fetching.

A week later I went with him to see the urologist. The treatment options were either surgery, or massive amounts of radiation, both of which would cause incontinence and impotence, at least for six months to two years, possibly for the rest of his life, the doctor said.

Our sex life was already so sparse—it had been half a year since we made love—how would this certain sentence of no intercourse affect us? When we found out about his cancer that night at the restaurant, I had resorted to humor, always my first line of defense.

"Well, that lets you off the hook," I said. "Way to go, dude!"

We laughed. But I was wincing inside.

The term prostate is so close to the word prostrate—to lay oneself flat on the ground in obeisance, to worship at the feet of a god, or an emperor.

We studied diagrams in a health education video. The prostate gland appeared as an upside-down triangle with a pointy end at the bottom. It sat right under the bladder.

The diagram showed cancer cells multiplying out of control, invading the prostate. Once you cut out the prostate—or radiate it—you kill cancer, but you also destroy or damage the nerves, shown in navy blue on the diagram, and that meant Lars would be wetting his pants and not able to have an erection for months, maybe years.

Later, we took a walk. Lars was quiet, more so than usual.

I said, "Honey, what's wrong?"

"I'm being hard on myself," he confessed, "I wonder if this cancer is my fault."

I stopped walking and turned to face him.

"When I got cancer, you didn't blame me. Don't blame yourself. It happens."

I squeezed his hand. We kept walking.

The diagrams and doctor visits and videos hadn't told us how to gin up our courage.

Fuck you, cancer! I thought. I beat it with surgery and no further treatment. Would Lars do the same? Why did lightning strike twice?

I wanted to believe the surgeon could spare the nerves around my husband's prostate so that he and I could escape the worst of the side effects. In the video, it showed how they reconnect the urethra once the prostate is gone. They sew it to the bladder. Scar tissue will form.

Scar tissue, that's what cancer left behind, and more. The big slap in the face. The bugle call to your mortality. Fear can prostrate you, and make you bow down to the god of death, to the underworld, to your disappearance.

No wonder Lars blamed himself. That was easier than letting death get a toe in the door. You have to be willing to fight cancer. I had been. But I wasn't sure about my husband. In the end, though, it was up to him.

I woke at 4 o'clock in the morning. Sleep eluded me. I snuggled deeper in our nest of sheets feeling the heat radiating from my husband's body, listening for his breath. I wasn't going to wake him. If I did, I'd have to say all the things I was afraid to say: *I'm terrified of losing you. I don't care if this is a treatable cancer, it's still cancer, and besides, something will kill you eventually. Just don't let it be now!*

I didn't want to admit that Lars seemed like the first truly dependable man I've ever been with, at least for our day-to-day routine. I had come to depend on him for so much that seemed mundane. Fixing things. Driving us places. Brainstorming. Walking along the rim of the hills hand-in-hand watching the light leach and then concentrate, the clouds the color of apricot jam. He had grown to be the butter to my bread, as Stanley Tucci told Meryl Streep in *Julie and Julia*.

"Lars, you are the butter to my bread," I tried to imagine myself telling him. Instead, I curled up next to him, mute, pretending to sleep as he sighed and turned over. He slept like a man who does not have a life-threatening disease, who does not have a terrified wife at his side, who does not even realize he is mortal.

Thank God you are not a complainer, I wanted to tell him, even though his obtuse cheerfulness drove me mad—it was better than the opposite. So much remained unspoken between us. I was afraid to be vulnerable, to tell him how much I cared. I was scared he couldn't or wouldn't reciprocate. I'd be left standing there with my desolate heart, exposed.

I joined a support group for spouses of cancer patients. Dealing with my husband's diagnosis was driving me over the edge. At one of our meetings, a member who was backlit on the Zoom screen so I couldn't see her face talked about her brother who had advanced stomach cancer and had decided on assisted suicide. I was coloring an intricate mandala to keep myself grounded in my chair rather than jumping up to run around the room screaming. "Suicide! Holy God! Is that where this cancer diagnosis is leading?"

I stared at the blurry woman. She wanted no such thing. She wanted him to keep getting chemo, to stay alive, to cope. She was willing to help him. But her sisters thought he should be allowed to kill himself. She had opened six months of back mail for him; she sorted the bills and the cancellation notices. His driver's license had expired. He hadn't paid his taxes. With each piece of reported procrastination, my breath got shallower. By the end, I was hyperventilating.

I wanted to cry for this woman, for her family, for all the ways cancer shattered them.

"Dear God," I prayed, "Please don't let that happen to us."

CHAPTER 27
ABBY

Sometimes the gods give us gifts. In a moment of desperation, one came to me in the shape of a very large dog.

My friend Dick, who leads our meditation group, was taking care of a Goldendoodle named Abby because her owner had had a stroke. When he mentioned this at the end of one of our Zoom meditations, I knew I wanted to meet her.

"I need some doggie love," I said. "Can I help you walk Abby?"

Worrying about which treatment Lars would choose for his cancer weighed on me. Surgery or radiation? Whatever he chose, would it be in time? He had procrastinated for many months. The clock was ticking.

Lars became almost comatose under stress. I was a hyperactive Jack in the Box. Day after day, we brushed past each other in our snug kitchen without speaking. We were so keyed up in our opposite ways that we weren't connecting at all. I was terrified and love-starved.

All beings crave the adoring gaze. Mothers bestow it on newborn babies. Lovers while making love. Dogs for any reason.

Dogs love without judgment or demands, without expectations. I was thirsty for that kind of unconditional love. I made a beeline toward Abby.

The moment she looked at me with her liquid brown eyes and snuffled her muzzle into my outstretched palm as if we had known each other forever, I knew her heart was with me. I bent down to her shaggy face.

"Oh Abby, what a good doggie ... what a sweet girl, what a lovey puppy dog." I burbled. She wagged her magnificent plume of a tail.

Abby was thirteen, anything but a puppy, but she had an innocence and sweetness that could melt the cold heart of the Grinch. She still loved to chase her tail and catch the ball.

Abby instinctively mirrored her humans while asking little of us—a pat on the head, a scoop of kibble, a kind word, a short walk. It was easy to fall in love with her.

Lars and I shared our wildly different stress responses, why not share the love?

"Would you like to meet Abby?"

"Sure," he said.

For once, I drove. We parked under a huge oak outside the dog park. We could hear the barking even before we opened the car doors, and once we did, it was a cacophony of tones from A minor to F sharp, and of voices from bass (the chocolate-colored hound) to soprano (the teacup poodles).

I immediately picked out Abby. She watched the little dogs like a gentle giant, taller than the others, and much calmer. A silent statue, golden and radiant.

I pointed. "That's Abby," I said.

Dick came over and shook hands with Lars. Abby trotted to our side. To my surprise, she nuzzled up to Lars first, and he bent down to pet her.

Lars had a way with animals. They were drawn to his calm, his silence, and his ability to sit for hours without moving.

Then Abby turned to me. She stood majestically as a lion, surveying her territory. I sank my hands deep into the golden mass of her thick wavy coat, scratched behind her ears, and crooned my unending song of *good dog, good dog, what a lovey girl, lovey dog, Abbykins, Abby my love.* Then reached in my pocket.

Abby cocked her head as if she not only knew what was on offer but wanted to thank me before I even extended my palm with half of a Milkbone biscuit. Her tail swished back and forth like a metronome. She was a radiant ball of life, her eyes locked with mine, my main squeeze.

The psychologist who led my Zoom support group for neuro-typical partners of people with Asperger's traits, wore a chunky orange necklace and a silk scarf. She looked like any woman of a certain age casually but elegantly put together. I had graduated from my cancer support group to one for non-autistic spouses of (mostly) husbands on the spectrum.

She explained that Aspies, as she called them, are strictly transactional. They just want to get stuff done. They don't understand the neurotypical way of relating to others. To them, feelings are insubstantial and unnecessary as fluff.

"Don't expect your Aspie to listen to your feelings, or even attempt to understand," she said. "They are experts at shutting down communication."

The autistic person will often say "I understand" simply to close the discussion. The others in their Zoom boxes nodded. It was a revelation to hear these other participants—mostly women—talk about their autistic husbands and boyfriends. I simultaneously realized that I was not alone, but also that I had been way off track trying to explain how I felt to my husband. I had been barking up the wrong tree, unlike Abby. She accepted people just as they were.

Lars dozed in the red leather chair as our ginormous Maine Coon cat sat on his belly. Marlowe was the captain of the Good Ship Lars, sailing on the waves of my husband's breath. The two of them—both large examples of the male species—seemed blissfully unaware of practical matters like what's for dinner.

But dog-loving neurotypical highly anxious me cared a lot about dinner. I was hungry for food and starving for connection.

I had made apple braised chicken in the slow cooker the night before. I went to the kitchen and pulled the leftovers out of the fridge. When I shut the door, I saw a photo of Abby held in place with refrigerator magnets, and a dry tickle began at the back of my throat.

I set the glass dish on the counter. I ran my finger over the outline of Abby's big body.

Marlowe sauntered in. He never missed a fridge door opening. Lars rustled out of the chair, the hum of its electric motor lowering the footrest to the floor, and although I couldn't see him, I felt him. A flare of anger rushed up my chest along with the gathering tears.

I opened the fridge again and gathered broccoli and salad makings.

Through the chopping, the cooking, the microwaving, I held tears at bay.

At last, I set two steaming plates on the table. Marlowe jumped up on the sideboard to watch us eat, and hunger outstripped my grief. I cut my food carefully, neat quarter inches of broccoli stalks, precise slices of chicken.

Lars put his head down to his plate and sucked in his breath on each bite as if he were slurping soup. I averted my eyes.

The silence was deafening. Earlier a neighbor had come over and Lars had chatted her up for twenty minutes. Now he sat there silent as a monument. I felt frozen. I did not know how to break through.

Talking about feelings was useless, using the language I knew how to speak. I needed some other way to reach him. But what was it?

Lars came and stood next to me as I was drying my hair one morning. I set down the hairdryer, grateful for a break from styling. He stopped by my left shoulder and leaned in for a peck on the lips. I was grateful for even a morsel. Like getting the last half teaspoon of jam from the bottom of the jar.

"I'm pondering," he said. I waited. Nothing more forthcoming?

"About what?" I asked.

"I had a sex dream," he said. "For the first time in a year."

Then he passed by me and clumped down the hall to his office, the bifold door squeaked as he shut it. Then it snapped back like an open fly in a pair of jeans. The contents of his disheveled office spilled into view.

I didn't ask for clarification. He was thinking about it, and I knew it would be days, if ever, before he would talk about it. Especially something as radioactive as our non-existent sex life. I had become "Aspergated," as autism expert Tony Atwood describes the spouses of ASD people. We learn to behave like our autistic loved one to defend against the pain.

I picked up the hairdryer again, grateful for the white noise. Did this mean he would want to make love again? Had the hormone shots he had received to suppress his testosterone worn off? Or maybe it was my diatribe last night. I had gathered my courage and told him that he wasn't doing his share, that he seemed disengaged, and he wasn't "taking care of our puppy," as our therapist Jonathan used to say.

We stopped seeing Jonathan. It had become too expensive, and all my energy was funneled into dealing with Lars's prostate cancer. The night before, I'd had a breakdown of sorts.

"The puppy is over there whimpering in the corner," I had said after dinner. I even pointed to the spot under the dining room window where our imaginary puppy was lying, dehydrated, with matted fur, barely alive. Lars looked blank, but he held my gaze.

"I need you to help me take care of the puppy," I said.

He got up and came around to my side of the table. He helped me out of my chair. He took me in his arms and gave me a long hug, patting my shoulder. I relaxed into him as best I could, not daring to hope.

"Are there any words that go with this hug?" I asked.

"Not right now," he said. And that was it.

Then this morning, the small hint that he was thinking about sex. He had finally decided on his treatment: he would get two kinds of radiation.

I called Dick and made a date to meet him at the dog park. I was desperate to see Abby.

CHAPTER 28
AUTISM

"What's going on with Lars?" Kate paused, "What's changed?"

She was calling from Portland. A lot had happened since our last call. Lars had had one intense session of brachytherapy, radiation delivered directly to his cancerous tumors, followed by three weeks of external beam radiation. That was early in November. We wouldn't know for sure if Lars was in remission until he had his first post-treatment PSA test in February.

Kate's mom had died in December, a few weeks before Christmas.

We were both grappling with the aftershocks in January.

I could hear Kate's twin boys in the background, dumping their tennis rackets in the hall, and heading to the kitchen for a snack. The pleasant yet annoying rustle of teenagers. For a moment, I wished I still had one. Then I realized, I did: my husband.

"It's not that Lars has changed," I said. "He's the same. Grumpy, depressed, not speaking to me. Sitting across the dinner table like a statue, rigid and silent."

"Mm-mm hmmm," she said. "That must be hard."

"Unbearable," I said. "What's changed is me. I am finally confronting what it means to live with someone who has a developmental disability."

In my support group for neurotypical partners of people with "Asperger's profiles" I've learned new things. Terms like "context blindness" and "impaired executive function," and "pervasive demand avoidance," a form of Oppositional Defiant Disorder. Autism often includes more challenges than just processing and talking about feelings.

"You think he has a disability?"

I can hear her multitasking, drawers sliding open, silverware clanking, trying to be sure her boys get food without destroying her kitchen.

"Yes," I said. "Autism is a pervasive developmental disorder. His brain does not work like ours. And that shows up in his behavior."

I tried to tamp down my panic, like banking a scorching fire. I soothed myself by rocking back and forth on the balls of my feet, my phone tucked into my pocket, my earbud cords strung across my chest.

"I'm married to a man whose brain function is not just different. It's impaired. He's brilliant when it comes to his special interests, but for emotions, or intimacy, or managing finances it's a non-starter. He thinks in a very different way."

Something else had changed. Kate didn't know about Abby. It turned out that Abby did not have glaucoma in one eye, as I thought because that's what Dick told me. She had a carcinoma in her brain. She stopped eating at the end of the first week of January. Soon, she couldn't move or control her bowels. Dick called a vet to come to the house and euthanize her.

I paced my kitchen and stopped to look at Abby's picture pinned to the fridge door.

I was with her when she died in Dick's living room. I whispered my goodbyes, told her what a good dog she was, how much she had helped me, and how thankful I was.

"I love you so much, Abby," I had whispered, laying my head on the floor next to hers. "Please watch over me."

I lit a candle I had brought. I set a vase of flowers on the coffee table. Abby deserved a dignified send-off. We arranged ourselves in a circle around her limp body.

After the vet administered the second injection, her big golden body grew stiff. The room was eerily quiet. Silently, I blew out the candle. I left the vase and the flowers for Dick.

Through my phone, I could hear the twins banging cupboard doors, slamming around Kate's kitchen. I'd never seen it, but I could imagine it—tall white cabinets, a big island, a double-wide fridge.

"I'm on the *phone*," she said to her sons, that edge of mother annoyance in her voice, at the same time the indulgence, the pleading, the forgiveness already granted.

"Just a minute," she said to me, "I'm going into the other room."

I let out my held breath. I was grateful I didn't have teenagers at home, only my big sulky husband, with the impulse control of a middle schooler and the same sweet clueless innocence as Kate's two sons.

But the difference between us was that Kate had an idea of what she would face ahead of time. She knew it the day she phoned me at work to tell me tests showed she was carrying twins. We both cried although she couldn't hear me—I'm good at suppressing tears.

"I just wanted a girl," she wailed on her end.

They already had a son, a demanding toddler, and now she was carrying two boys. I felt proud of her. How she had adjusted and raised her family, carrying a heavier load.

I didn't know ahead of time what would be required of me with an autistic partner, or how Lars would change when he had lost the motivation to mask his autism. Of course, I knew he was quirky. That he had mood swings. That he saw things differently. I even suspected he might have ASD-1 (formerly Asperger's). Like many partners of older men, because Lars had gone through life undiagnosed, I was the one to suggest he was autistic.

I had convinced myself I could handle it, that if I was patient and offered lots of physical touch and reassurance, we'd be able to bridge our differences. For a while, it worked.

"I'm back," she said, a bit breathless. "So, you were saying …"

"I am in pain," I said. "Kate, I am in so much pain."

The Australian comedian Hannah Gadsby says that people with post-traumatic stress disorder and people on the autism spectrum have a lot in common. In her 2019 TED talk "Three Ideas. Three Contradictions. Or Not." she said this: "I began to think a lot about how PTSD and autism have so much in common and I started to worry—because I have both."

While I couldn't know for sure whether Lars had PTSD, I knew that I did. I suspected he was neurodivergent but since he refused to be evaluated, I didn't know that for sure either. What I did know is that while many of our characteristics expressed differently, they also overlapped. We were both highly sensitive and easily overwhelmed. We both suffered from toxic shame and harsh inner critics. We both liked to disappear through hyper-focus into a great piece of art, a good book, a beautiful film, or surrender to the rhythm of dance music.

Humor was a strength for both of us, yet we were both overly serious at times. Both of us could get down in the weeds with details. We were both outstanding at completing tasks and we often procrastinated. When stressed beyond endurance, we both had meltdowns. My flight instincts were easily triggered; Lars would more naturally freeze and shut down.

Bottom line: we were both vulnerable. To protect ourselves, we masked our "differability," our special ways of soothing ourselves.

A book I read on the mysteries of love between different neurotypes written by Rudy Simone, said this: "One day you feel as if your relationship is finally on solid ground, and the next day that ground has dropped out from under you."

As an abuse survivor with complex grief, having the ground shift in my intimate relationship was profoundly disturbing. And yet that's what I unknowingly signed up for when I married Lars.

"Women in love with Asperger men tend to be smart capable women who like a challenge in a relationship. But even so, it may be more of a challenge at times than you bargained for," Simone wrote.

Kate had caught me on one of those days, a day of shifting sands, when the challenge of being married to Lars seemed unendurable.

When I say Lars is kind but not empathetic, some people look puzzled. How does that work, exactly? Here's an example: Lars will open car doors, carry grocery bags, go to Costco in search of some obscure item I might want, say Britta filters, or help a neighbor on the spur of the moment with a frazzled computer. But if I say I feel sad, or upset, or angry about something he'll look into space. He won't draw me out, ask questions, or nod sagely as I speak. He will be mystified. He may space out or ignore me altogether.

The night the Caldor fire jumped Echo Ridge in the horrible fire summer of 2021, I stood next to our bed, weeping inconsolably.

Lars was in bed, earbuds plugged in, one hand against his temple like The Thinker.

"Can you talk?" I stood there, bereft.

He cracked open one eye, then the other. He pulled out both earbuds.

"Tahoe, the lake, the forests, the mountains—it's all going up in smoke."

The tears came.

"All that ash going into the lake," I sobbed.

He waited, said nothing, and stared past me. I had just delivered my aria to an empty auditorium. When I'd finally cried all I could, and climbed into bed, he put a hand on my shoulder and held me in place as if I might blow away.

Whenever we got into a tight spot, our past breakup loomed. When we reunited, Lars had sworn he would never walk away, almost as if by having done it once, he would never have to do it again. Breakup as a gesture. But I suspected he had moments of wanting to flee. I certainly did.

During my freak out over his cancer diagnosis, when it seemed that he would never choose a treatment option and we'd be swirling in a hell of indecision until his cancer metastasized and grew like a fungus into his bones, I plummeted into anticipatory grief. He might die! My overhyped type A brain/body drew this conclusion: If he's going to leave me, I'll leave him first!

Part of what drove me so crazy about the first time he broke up with me is that I did not initiate it. It blindsided me. I didn't get to choose. His cancer landed the same way.

"How dare you get cancer?" I wanted to yell at him.

Of course, I'd had cancer myself the year before. I was furious at myself too.

At least I was an equal-opportunity control freak. Even though part of me knew better, I wanted to believe that life was predictable. But as the many experts I'd read on autism pointed out, being married to a neurodivergent spouse meant living with the unexpected. You had to be willing to be surprised over and over, and not necessarily in a good way.

CHAPTER 29
DAY TO DAY

May of 1955. I am about to turn seven. I've never had a real party for my birthday. My family celebrates with a family dinner, some cake, and a few presents. But I want more! I dream of a surprise birthday party with all the trimmings. When I ask my mother, she says no.

So, I begin my campaign.

"All my friends have surprise parties."

"Just this one time, please."

"Please, please, please."

Finally, Mom gives in.

On the afternoon of the party, the dining room table is piled with wrapped boxes with ribbons because gift bags aren't a thing yet. Balloons float around the room. A "Pin the Tail on the Donkey" made of thin cardboard is tacked to the closet door: a beige donkey and some yellow straw. We each get blindfolded and spun around, then stagger toward the door, holding out our beige tails with thumbtacks in them to pin on the donkey.

May of 2022. I discovered that my sister thinks that Mom planned the party. Tess called to wish me a happy seventy-fourth birthday and mentioned how jealous she was because our mother had thrown a party for me.

"No way," I said. "I lobbied like crazy for that party."

We talked about how hard I worked to engineer my own birthday celebration.

Lars overheard this conversation, at least tangentially, because we were in the car. I told him how my mother would never have planned a kid's party on her own.

"Having hosted a lot of them over the years, I can't say I blame her," I mused.

I flashed back over the parties I planned for Maya and Greta, the gift bags, the excited squeals of eight little girls, the hot dogs, and juice boxes.

"I don't regret any of those parties," I said, remembering my children's sweet, excited faces with cake smeared on their cheeks, how good it felt to make them happy.

We were in his car driving to Sebastopol for my birthday celebration, meeting Greta and Jim and the girls at a local winery for a tasting, and then going out to dinner.

At that moment, I realized the glaring truth: I had engineered this family gathering too. Lars didn't lift a finger. I was still running my deeply grooved program of taking charge, making myself responsible for everything turning out okay.

I was reading *Oh William* by Elizabeth Strout. Lucy Barton comes to the end of the story not knowing her ex-husband, although she knows him better than anyone. Everyone is a mystery. Even us, even our younger selves.

For my birthday, Lars got me a dark chocolate candy bar and a card he picked off the rack at our neighborhood CVS drug store. The verse on the card said: "Your friendship has planted a little garden in my heart."

On the front, there's a picture of a little girl watering a gigantic flower with birds perched on the petals; the flower centers are made of colored plastic beads, blue, yellow, and pink, which match the little birds. The watering spout sprinkles shiny blue confetti on the ground at the flowers' roots.

It would have been the perfect card for my seventh birthday.

"I didn't sign up for a life of celibacy, Lars. You say we should schedule sex. But you'd be doing it only because I wanted to, not because you do."

Lars was holding back tears, red-rimmed eyes staring at me.

"That's one step away from paying for it!"

I had tried to modulate my voice at first, but now I'd lost it. My words were projectiles; I was raining verbal bombs on his head.

Where was the calm reasoned voice who understood both sides? The one who could bring us together? Now that we had quit therapy with Jonathan, we no longer had a mediator.

We faced off over the dining room table, two warring countries, each with its grievances, its boundaries, its weather. I was a typhoon lashing at my silent husband. Lars was a humid Midwest afternoon right before a thunderstorm, the held back rain, the growing pressure, the barometer falling. I wished I could be a tropical island, with the scent of hibiscus and jasmine in the lush night air.

I'm speaking my truth, but it's a truth that's too loud, a truth he can't hear. I see it in the unshed tears, his slumping shoulders, and the way he looks like a defiant five-year-old.

In a couples' communication class we took on Zoom, we learned that anger is considered a secondary emotion; one we use to avoid deeper feelings. Beneath anger is always emotional pain, our instructor said. A click went off in my head. I decided to let myself go all the way to the bottom of an ocean of pain.

*

"I am in pain," I said, holding back tears.

"Mm-hmm," Lars said. We were lying in bed, the sun just rising outside our window.

"I am in so much pain," I said again. "I am lost."

I had learned not to expect an answer or even a supportive comment. I was still smarting from the last-minute birthday gift, the wildly inappropriate card.

I threw off the covers, got dressed, and took the dog we were watching for a vacationing friend for a walk.

The dog, a rescued poodle mix, pranced like a cartoon poodle, like a dog you imagine walking down the street in Paris with a fashionable lady holding its diamond-studded leash. I was not that. I was dressed in sweats walking a prancing poodle at 6:30 in the morning, wearing a black baseball cap pulled over my messy hair, attempting to soothe my pain.

If there is an arc to this story it's like a doodle made by a manic depressive. Hope, despair, hope, anger, hope, grave disappointment, hope, trying again, more frustrated hope. It's an unending graph of unresolved conflict, an unopened love letter, a colossal disconnect.

*

Put ice cubes in the orchid pots. Change the burnt-out bulb in the bathroom. Clean the cat box. Bring in a package of chicken breasts from the garage refrigerator. Cancel our plans for the baseball game. *Did you? Will you? Please. Thank you.*

It's time to go. Lars is driving. He's carried all the luggage to the car, including the crinkly blue Ikea bag with my two pillows, a small fan, and my windbreaker, scarf, and gloves, in case it's cold at the coast. Pigeon Point can be windy. I packed two turtlenecks, flannel pajamas, a couple of sweaters, and my new hiking boots.

I gave my husband instructions. They mapped to the instructions I gave myself. Parallel lines. I packed the luggage. He carried it. I put the food in the garage fridge, he retrieved it. I planned the trip, he will drive. Logistics are our forte.

"Did you leave the porch light on?"

"Did you close the windows?"

"Did you remember your water bottle?"

"Did you bring pretzels?"

You might imagine we're prepping for a two-week road trip. But no. It's just two days in a wooden cabin overlooking the hills and trees with a porch swing on the deck, a hot tub at the lodge, and a sauna at the "comfort station" where the showers and sinks are.

I wished for a comfort station in my marriage, a place where we each could go to be wrapped in a cozy blanket and soothed by wiser beings, maybe our grandparents or great grandparents. Mine would speak to me in French, and sing "Alouettes" or "Sur le Pont D'Avignon." Lars's ancestors would whisper "Jeg elsker deg" and sing Norwegian lullabies.

But comforting ourselves was an inside job. We were stumbling up a very steep hill, our learning curve as a couple with different neurotypes stretched in front of us. If only there was a neat way to end this part of the story. But life is messy. Beautiful, but full of loose ends.

CHAPTER 30
STUFF I LEFT OUT REDUX

1. I hate writing about sex. It's too easy to drop into cliché, or over describing. It's hard to get to the heart of the matter because it's less about physical details, and more about intangibles like desire, self-esteem, and the complex workings of the brain. I hesitate. There's Lars. Then there's me. And a stew of aging issues. We are both cancer survivors. Recovery takes time. I hate the stereotypes that label sex in older people as somehow humorous or adorable, but aberrant. How people laugh about older people having sex, how amusing it is to read about the rates of herpes in nursing homes, and how old bodies gross us out. I was that way too when I was younger; the thought of crepe-y skin and flaccid penises horrified me. But it's not so gross when it's all you have. Penetration may be out of reach, but foreplay still feels amazing.

2. The Palace of Fine Arts in San Francisco is a red sandstone Greco-Roman temple constructed for the 1915 Panama-Pacific exposition. We went there to see the Australian comedian Hannah Gadsby, who happens to be autistic, and who appeared on stage with two fake rabbits, one lit

from within. You don't know why the rabbits are there until the penultimate scene where Gadsby recounts her proposal of marriage to her lady love and producer Jenny or "Jen-o," as Gadsby calls her. Gadsby clues us in early about her proposal of marriage being somewhat unconventional, about how they had had a "team meeting" beforehand to discuss it. Sitting there in row J, seats 54 and 56, Lars had his hand on my knee. He gave me a little squeeze. Most marriage proposals are "reverse engineered spontaneity," she said. Ours certainly was, given that I was coaching him on what to say beforehand and taking him to purchase a ring I'd already picked out. Gadsby has a lot to say about her relationship with neurotypical Jen-O. It's funny as hell and very wise. I felt less alone hearing it, knowing that Jen-O was there off stage, cheering Hannah on, capably managing every detail.

3. In Chapter 10, I told you I was "wealth adjacent," living close to people whose economic means surpass mine. Does that make me a privileged twit? Or am I a person with a strong urge for self-preservation in a culture that is rapidly plummeting to new spiritual, political, and economic lows? I used to have qualms about my status as an aging diva in a cossetted retirement community far from the madding crowd. As a young single mother, Maya and I subsisted on food stamps. I barely made the rent each month. I applied for Medicaid. Maya wore hand-me-downs until I got a corporate job and started making real money. She stole clothes from Macy's and Nordstrom in high school because I could not afford to keep up with wealthier parents and she was determined to. I was better able to support Greta because by the time

she cared about Nordstrom I'd been making real money for several years. Now I'm one of those greedy Boomers you read about who are busy depleting the Social Security Trust Fund and spending our children's inheritances.

4. My mother left my grandmother's five-bedroom house on Lake Erie to her partner of twenty-six years, Cecile. Mom left the contents to her three kids. With the help of an appraiser, we worked it out and Tess, Tim, and I each got a few thousand bucks. Lars's parents left their home to his sister. He never got a penny. He would say this is fair given that Kristen, who is a nurse, looked after their parents in their declining years and never moved farther than a few towns away as an adult. Lars left New York state and never looked back, and rarely talked to his family until the final years of his parents' lives. We were both disinherited. Going it alone emotionally and economically is challenging. We both survived, but the experience left scars.

5. Talking honestly about autism is a risk. First of all, there's still a stigma attached. Second, even experts in the field don't always agree on its parameters, or the language to use. Third, autistic people are getting pretty pissed off about neurotypical people attempting to define them. In writing about Lars, I'm walking a line. I'm telling a story about a mixed marriage between two people with different neurotypes. In doing that, I'm biased in favor of my own experience, while also trying to recount his as fairly as I can. I don't pretend to speak for him. I can only speak for myself.

6. Autism researcher Simon Baron-Cohen, a professor of developmental psychology at Trinity College, Cambridge,

argues that autism is both a disability and a difference. He advocates for providing support for the disability while at the same time valuing the difference. It is vital to avoid "sledgehammer" approaches, finding a cure for autism, or forcing autistic people into the mold of the neurotypical world, he says.

7. Renowned animal behaviorist Temple Grandin has speculated that if autism were eliminated, society would lose most of its scientists, musicians, and mathematicians. Diagnosed as an adult, Grandin was one of the first to publicly disclose that she was autistic. Her book *The Autistic Brain: Thinking Across the Spectrum* discusses her life experiences and how advances in technology have revolutionized the understanding of autism and its connection to the brain.

8. At Hannah Gadsby's "A Body of Work" show in San Francisco, she mentioned her diagnosis of autism. A group in the front row cheered loudly. "My people," Gadsby said, turning to bow in their direction. Then, turning back to the entire audience, she said she could guarantee there were many more people with ASD in the theater. She considers her diagnosis a positive because it gave her a framework for understanding her struggles, and her feelings of isolation; it challenged her belief that she was somehow just a messed-up person doing messed-up things. She wondered aloud what her life might have been like had she been diagnosed earlier. I wonder the same thing about Lars.

9. I loved Lars and he drove me crazy. But I also drove myself crazy. As he used to say, "It's not a very long drive."

10. If all I ever got to do for the rest of my life was snuggle in our big bed with my husband, chop vegetables together in our cozy kitchen, take walks around the Rossmoor golf course, and sit together in the evening reading or watching TV, it might have been enough. I was willing to sacrifice for the sake of companionship. I had hoped that we would make peace with ourselves and each other. In the beginning I believed that we would stay together "until death do us part," just like we promised on our wedding day. It is proving very difficult to let go of that dream.

CHAPTER 31
UNENDING

"Is this a Rhumba or a Fox Trot?"

"Not sure. Shall we dance anyway?"

"Okay."

Lars took my hand and led me out to the dance floor. The men wore dark suits, and the women festive cocktail dresses and sparkly jewelry. It was a far cry from our Zydeco nights at Eagles when we wore jeans and cowboy boots. I had been nervous about going to a dinner dance at the Rossmoor Event Center. It seemed so old school. How do you eat a three-course meal and dance at the same time?

When the music began, my husband led me expertly. True, it was not the bluesy down and dirty sway of Zydeco, but ballroom dancing has a rhythm and elegance all its own. Lars beamed down at me with his effervescent smile.

During the salad course, we did the Fox Trot. After eating our pasta, we waltzed. We did a made-up version of the Rhumba with Zydeco overtones after the main course. And when the four-piece band struck up a Polka, I couldn't resist. Growing up in Cleveland alongside Italians and Croatians, I'd learned to Polka. It came as naturally as skipping. My feet barely touched the floor as Lars spun me around.

"Stop! I'm so dizzy," I pleaded, panting. He kept going.

Finally, I rebelled and stood still. Lars spun me into an open skaters hold, and we sashayed back to our table keeping time to the music.

I sat in my chair sweating, my head spinning, just like in the old days. Only this time, a server brought a piece of cake to the table and sat it down at my place. Dessert!

Our table of eight danced, and ate, and drank too much wine. I watched as seventy and eighty-year-olds made their moves with panache, envious of some of the more skillful dancers. They looked so elegant! When I went to the restroom to freshen up, a woman told me she admired my Polka dancing. I laughed with pleasure and said thank you.

My steps had grown light as dandelion down. I was floating. Lars was solid as ever, and so graceful. Our dancing filled me with hope.

That night would be the last time we danced together, but I didn't know that at the time. We moved together as one body, both happy, both drawn back into the magic circle of two we made when we danced.

I fell into bed that night happy and exhausted. Within minutes, I was sound asleep.

It was pitch black when I felt a little squirrel paw on my left breast kneading my skin through my pajama top. I cracked an eyelid. The clock read 2:00, its blinking red numerals glowed. The slight pawing continued. I smiled and went back to sleep.

At 5:00 o'clock, the squirrel paw reappeared more urgently. Lars pressed against me, and I felt his erection. He held me against his body with both arms.

Be careful what you pray for, I thought.

I wasn't sure I remembered how. It had been so long. I pushed back against him, and he began to kiss my neck, and then my back. When he wedged his hand between my thighs I opened them. He tugged at my hair, arching my head back. We were on again!

"Dancing is foreplay," one friend said. Apparently, she was right.

Lars carried on in his methodical way, working his way down my body. He brought me to a thumping orgasm with his mouth and tongue just as skillfully as before. I was delirious.

But when I tried to stroke his penis, he said it hurt.

"Show me how," I begged. "You can ask for anything, and I'll give it to you. Tell me what you want."

He only laughed.

"I don't know what I want," he said.

I knew better than to press for answers.

I snuggled into him. His chest hairs tickled my nose. I listened to his breath deepen and slow. I thought of Ed and Nids in their kitchen kissing. I drifted. When I opened my eyes again, the clock said 8:00, and his side of the bed was empty.

After we had made love again, it seemed like a miracle. There was hope!

The next night, I lit a votive candle, and filled the bathtub full of lavender-scented bubbles. I set the candle holder I gave Lars the first Christmas we were dating on the side of the tub, and climbed in, remembering how he had casually tucked it back in its gift box. It meant little to him. It was just candlelight, unconnected to romance or seduction.

Later, I had discovered that he didn't like any light in the bedroom during sex. I learned to be happy making love with him in the dark and the candle holder migrated to the bathtub.

I sank up to my neck in bubbles and watched as indentations in the Mercury glass cast shadows on the bathroom tile. They flickered and danced, a macrame of light, lacey and beautiful. Comforting.

I had intended the candle holder to be an invitation. I thought it would communicate my willingness to become his lover. But now I wondered. Maybe I didn't know any more than Lars did what it actually meant. The flame wavered and danced, the way our relationship flickered on and off. All along, perhaps I should have focused on the candle flame, not the holder.

Hypnotized by the flickering candle, I let myself dream. Maybe one day I'd take the candle holder and restore it to our bedside table, a talisman of lessons learned, of all the ways we met each other beyond words.

When it burned out I'd put another candle in its place. It would be like the eternal flame, a marker of our heroic effort. It would flicker and burn the way the words of our different languages scraped against each other so that one meaning ignited another.

It would be like the Tower of Babel, a place where the languages of the world collided, where the autistic mind met the allistic one to forge a new language. Except that in the Bible, God curses the tower builders to a permanent state of confusion and disconnection.

At that moment, I clung to my tattered hope. I still believed there was a chance for us; I was determined to keep trying. But I could not know how sorely I would be tested, or how unhappy Lars was. Our connection was increasingly tenuous.

Unvoiced resentments grew. The candle flamed out more often than before, and eventually sputtered out entirely.

It was a potent cycle of hope, disappointment, missed opportunities, and deep hurt.

EPILOGUE

I had been 5,000 miles away visiting friends in Switzerland to celebrate my 75th birthday. Halfway through my six-week trip, I wrote Lars a "love sandwich," a technique I learned from our autism coach during my sessions with her.

I told him I still loved him and wanted to save our marriage, and expressed hope that he did too. Then I asked three questions: Was he setting up individual coaching sessions? Did he still want to learn the communication and problem-solving process for neurodiverse couples? Did he still want to save our marriage? I ended the message by repeating that I loved him and hoped he would join me in trying to repair our relationship.

Two days of radio silence followed. In my heart, I knew.

"I'm recognizing that my behaviors demonstrate that I've withdrawn from our relationship, from our marriage," Lars wrote to me at last. He asked me to bear with his intellectualizing as he analyzed his thoughts. Then he wrote about an obscure sect of Catholic ascetics who re-enact the Stations of the Cross and whip themselves as a penance, the Penitentes.

I stared at the screen, trying to decipher the cryptic message embedded in his email. What did he mean? Did he view himself as a Penitente? He didn't explain.

He reminded me that when we had reunited after our four-year interregnum, he had promised himself he wouldn't take any actions when he was feeling down.

"Of course, withdrawal is an action in itself. And, if the funds were in the bank, I'd suggest we pay off these mortgages, buy me a place of my own, and see whether living together apart repairs our marriage," he added.

I agreed with him that withdrawing is an action. Frozen silence is a choice. A perpetual scowl sends a very strong message, one I took to heart. The message was, "Don't bother me."

"I do say that joining with you seemed like a good idea at the time," he concluded.

It had seemed like a good idea to me too five years ago when being together meant going to art museums and plays, traveling together on an Alaska cruise and to visit our siblings in Ohio and New York. We were dancing together then, sharing dinners out, discussing the latest articles in *The Atlantic* or *The New Yorker*. We were also having semi-regular sex and building an intimate emotional connection. Did I imagine that?

I wanted to ask, *What happened to the man I thought I married? Why did you turn into someone who would not even speak to me across the dinner table, let alone have sex with me?*

Several days passed. Then Lars wrote again.

"I think I would be happier if we lived separately."

"I think that's a good idea," I wrote back, tapping the keyboard with swift strokes.

I stared out the window drinking in the garden where I was staying in a district of Basel. It was late May. Climbing roses splashed crimson petals against the terrace wall, and butterflies feasted on a disorderly bed of lavender and buttercups, a nod to the nearby Jura Mountains, to the countryside where my hosts hiked on weekends.

I'd tried so hard to keep us together, to turn myself into a patient spouse who could tolerate the loneliness of an Asperger's marriage. Lars called the question. I answered honestly. I was exhausted, dispirited, clinging to the shreds of my identity. I no longer recognized myself. Being with dear ones in Switzerland snapped me back to myself. Only then could I acknowledge the toll the marriage had exacted.

Once I put an ocean between us, I could see how my attempts to help were backfiring. Lars didn't want my help. He didn't want me fixing dinner, managing our social calendar, or trying to set up a budget. He didn't want to talk about what wasn't working in our marriage. He wanted to sit in front of his computer screen, disappear into his digital black hole, and live free of gravity. Free of problems. Free of me and my neurotypical brain, and confusing feelings, the imperative E.M. Forster wrote in *Howard's End* to "only connect," exactly what he couldn't do. He wanted to be single. Autonomous. Whole within himself.

The moment I read his words I knew he was right.

The imperative was this: Leave me alone!

I wish I could be more "When Harry Met Sally" and less "Wuthering Heights." I desperately wanted our story to have a happy ending. I hoped the moments of laughter and connection would grow, and the communication misfires might lessen. After all our tribulations, I wanted to be one of the tenacious neurodiverse couples who finds a way to work it out.

Instead, our relationship crumbled like a sandcastle hit by a wave at high tide, leaving only the faintest outline behind. I had to accept the truth: Lars's primary need was for autonomy, while mine was for connection. We were pulling in opposite directions.

By the time I returned from Europe there was no relationship left to save. I had used up every ounce of energy and good will I had. There was very little left of the old me, either. We agreed to separate in June 2023. Later, I would learn that eighty-five percent of couples with mixed neurotypes eventually divorce. What we had attempted was exceedingly difficult.

By that point our occasional bursts of sexual intimacy had flamed out. Once I found an attorney and initiated the legal process, Lars disappeared into his office and began obsessively rearranging financial data in his QuickBooks. We stopped speaking. There would be no more dancing, even with a coatrack.

🧩

I shook with fear. I had just told my attorney, "File! I want a divorce!"

I drove to the freeway in a trance, barely seeing the trees lining Olympic Boulevard, the bicyclists in the bike lane, the other cars heading to Highway 24. The ground was dropping out from under me.

I called my sister.

"I have to save myself," I said, fighting back tears.

"Stay strong! You are doing the right thing," she said.

🧩

In one of the support groups for women attempting to leave their neurodivergent husbands that I still attend, the facilitator explained that men with ASD go into "divorce mode." Either they move and leave no forwarding address, don't respond to legal filings, and generally dodge any formal proceedings, or they become hyper focused on numbers, obsessively creating spreadsheets, and fighting with their estranged spouses over every stick of furniture and every shared penny.

When I announced that I had found an apartment to rent at Rossmoor, Lars only nodded. As I prepared to move, and divide our furniture, he refused to let me take an area rug I asked for. I reminded him that it actually belonged to my daughter. Then, he told me I couldn't take my motorized sit-stand desk because he had selected it online and paid for it with his credit card.

"Take the desk," my attorney advised.

"I'm just waiting for him to ask for the engagement ring back," I said.

"That's one of the few things in family law that's crystal clear," my lawyer said. "You get to keep the rings."

To cover myself, I took photos of every room in our house. Then I created a Word table with every lamp, pillow, and sofa cushion, whether it was community or separate property, and who would take it. I put my engagement ring back in its black velvet box and packed it with my other jewelry.

The six weeks we lived together while legally separated were like burning in Purgatory. When I discovered that Lars had given a private code, including the last four digits of my Social Security number, to a stranger, I lost it. I overheard this as he was talking on his phone. It was one more boundary violation in a seemingly endless string of them. When I challenged him, he went on a diatribe about how he had a perfect right to do it.

"I'm getting a new accountant," he explained. "He asked to view our return."

"Shut up! Just shut up!" I shouted, leaping to my feet.

"You are violating my privacy," I fumed. "Call our accountant and get your own fucking code!"

The next day, I booked an online moving service and did a partial move, taking only my desk, my mattress, some clothes, a few kitchen basics and books, and my cat Marlowe.

The following week, while Lars was seeing clients, I hired helpers and spent three frantic days packing boxes, returning at night to my new apartment to sleep. The moving company came at the end of the week and took the rest of my furniture, plants, art, and books. At last, I could breathe! I had secured a refuge.

The exercise pool at the Fitness Center buzzed like a beehive as we waited for water aerobics to begin. To warm up, I strode through the water, weaving between women bobbing on floaties. It's like this most Fridays—it's a popular class, easy on the joints, but a great workout.

As I faced the spot where the instructor stands, I felt a tap on my shoulder. When I turned, I saw a woman with short white hair, and a pretty shade of lipstick.

"I think you're beautiful," she said.

It was a jaw dropping moment.

"Oh, gosh," I stammered, "Thank you!"

It had been so long since anyone had told me I was beautiful. Or paid me any compliment at all. Or even spoke to me. I was living alone now. I talked to my cat.

"You have a great figure," she said.

"Gosh," I repeated. "Should we go on a lunch date?"

I covered my vulnerability with humor, my favorite hideout.

I thanked her again, then returned to my spot. But something made me turn and walk back to her.

"Honestly, I'm grateful to you," I said. "I'm going through a divorce. It's so painful. You don't know how much your kindness means to me."

"I'm sorry," she said. "Alcoholic?"

"Autistic," I said. "I just couldn't do it any longer."

She gave me a look that said, "I understand. I'm with you."

For a moment, sunlight burnished the water. Our eyes locked. I felt seen. I remembered the woman I had been before, the woman who was okay on her own, a breadwinner, a single mom. I imagined the woman I could become now, tougher, wiser, more aware that everything doesn't always work out in the end. A fish without a bicycle.

Up to my chest in water, I straightened my shoulders and walked back to my place, inhabiting myself again.

ACKNOWLEDGEMENTS

Gratitude to Ann Peterson, who first encouraged me to query Vine Leaves Press, and to Melanie Faith, who so deftly critiqued my submission, and offered editorial feedback and support throughout the process. For the many others at Vine Leaves Press who helped make this book a reality, including my fellow authors, thank you.

For the brave therapists and coaches who speak the languages of opposite neurotypes and support couples, often as they discover their neurodivergence, I'm in your debt. Special thanks to Sarah Swenson, LMHC, who wrote the foreword to this book and to Grace Myhill, MSW, who leads the Neurodiverse Couples Institute and provides support to countless people.

Much of *Disconnected* was first written in Elizabeth Stark's Advanced Craft Workshop in Zoom sessions during the pandemic. My sisters in that enterprise saved my sanity.

Thank you to my colleagues at the San Francisco Writers Grotto and Left Margin Lit who provided sanctuary and feedback as I rewrote the manuscript, offering encouragement when I needed it most. Special thanks to Kathy Seligman, Laurie Ann Doyle, and Louise Nayer for their insights.

To Dana Gaskin-Wenig and Sarah Scott Davis, your love, support and close reading keeps me at my desk. And to the many memoirists who write true, courageous stories, often at great personal risk, I stand on your shoulders.

For my friends and family, your love provided sustenance in the darkest hours. And for my estranged husband, the Lone Ranger of this story, what we had in the early years was magic. I'm sad that it didn't last.

RESOURCES FOR NEURODIVERSE COUPLES

The Other Half of Asperger Syndrome: A Guide to Living in an Intimate Relationship with a Partner Who is on the Autism Spectrum, 2nd edition, Maxine Aston, (Jessica Kingsley Publishers, 2014)

The Autism Couple's Workbook, 2nd edition, Maxine Aston (Jessica Kingsley Publishers, 2020)

The Complete Guide to Asperger's Syndrome, Tony Attwood (Jessica Kingsley Publishers, 2012)

22 Things a Woman Must Know If She Loves a Man with Asperger's Syndrome, Rudy Simone, (Jessica Kingsley Publishers, 2009)

Have they Gone Nuts? The Survival Guide to Social Interaction in Neurodiverse Relationships, Bronwyn M. Wilson, Ph.D., (Ultimate World Publishing, 2022)

Love and Asperger's: Practical Strategies to Help Couples Understand Each Other and Strengthen Their Connection, Kate McNulty, LCSW (Rockridge Press, 2020)

The Journal of Best Practices: A Memoir of Marriage, Asperger Syndrome, and One Man's Quest to be a Better Husband, David Finch (Scribner, 2012)

Find more at *eleanorvincent.com*

VINE LEAVES PRESS

Enjoyed this book?
Go to *vineleavespress.com* to find more.
Subscribe to our newsletter: